RECOVER YOUR HEALTH

Simple Uncensored Health Strategies

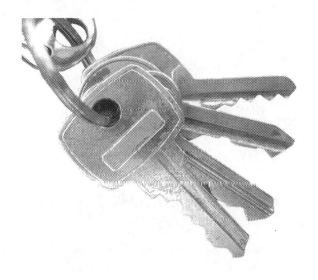

By

Dr. Jeremiah Joseph

BALBOA.
PRESS
A DIVISION OF HAY HOUSE

Balboa Press books may be ordered through booksellers or by contacting:

Balboa Press
A Division of Hay House
1663 Liberty Drive
Bloomington, IN 47403
www.balboapress.com
1-(877) 407-4847

ISBN: 978-1-4525-4974-3 (sc)
ISBN: 978-1-4525-4973-6 (e)

Balboa Press rev. date: 05/03/2012

TABLE OF CONTENTS

ACKNOWLEDGEMENTS

I dedicate this book, first to my beautiful and loving wife Kristin. The support and balance in our unwavering beliefs about health and the faith we share has allowed me to become the best doctor I can be. I can only pray that I can provide the same standards of encouragement, love and patience that you have instilled in me. You are a phenomenal doctor that has touched thousands of lives and you will unknowingly touch millions in the future with your brilliant mind.

To my son Josiah: Daddy loves you more than anything buddy. Know that mommy and I will do everything in our power to make sure that you grow up healthy, loved, and blessed. You have provided me with so much excitement for life and have shown me what unconditional love really is about.

To my parents, Darlene and Art: Most of my success comes from the deep-rooted foundational principles that have molded my life into what I am today. You have supported every decision that I have made since childhood whether right or wrong. There has never been a time in my life that you doubted me or were not there for me. For those things and so much more, I am forever grateful and love you.

Lastly, thank you to my mentors: Jim Rohn, Dr.'s Chris and Danielle Hood, Brian Tracy, David Singer, Dr. Deepak Chopra, and Harvey Diamond.

To my TEAM members in my clinics: your mission, purpose and eternal devotion to helping the sick avoid needless medications and surgeries will never go unnoticed.

DISCLAIMER AND NOTICES

The information and recommendations outlined in this book are not intended as substitutes for personalized medical advice; the reader of this book should see a qualified healthcare provider. This book proposes certain theoretical methods of nutrition and health that are not necessarily mainstream. It is the sole responsibility of the user of the information included in this book to determine if the procedures and recommendations described are appropriate. The author cannot be held responsible for any inadvertent errors or omissions in the information.

The information in this book should not be construed as a claim or representation that any procedure or product mentioned constitutes a specific cure, palliative, or ameliorative. Procedures and nutritional recommendations described should be considered as adjunctive to other conventional procedures deemed necessary by the attending licensed doctor.

It is the concern of the Department of Health and Human Services that no homeopathic or nutritional supplements replace established, conventional medical approaches, especially in cases of emergencies, serious or life–threatening diseases, or conditions. I share the concern, as replacing conventional treatment with such remedies, especially in serious cases, may deprive the patient of necessary treatment and thereby cause harm, and may pose a legal liability for the healthcare professional involved. The nutritional recommendations made in this book should not replace conventional medical treatment. The Food and Drug Administration has not evaluated the nutritional supplements or products in this book, and the supplements and or products are not intended to diagnose, treat, cure, or prevent disease.

THE SECRETS OF HAVING A SHARP MIND, CHILD-LIKE ENERGY AND THE FIERY WEIGHT-LOSS METABOLISM OF A TRACK ATHLETE

If you were to ask a group of people what they think "being healthy" is, most people will probably tell you that it's not feeling sick. But while not having any symptoms or diseases is one important aspect of health, there are other many other components that are equally as important. In fact, in 1947 the World Health Organization defined health as: "a state of complete physical, mental, and social well-being and not merely the absence of disease or infirmity."

Although true health is difficult to define, it is easy to achieve if you know how and have the right tools. At the end of the day, achieving and maintaining overall good health comes down to just four essentials—food, water, oxygen and nerve supply. And the relative importance of each of these essentials may surprise you.

> **Think About It:** You can survive without food for 40 days, without water for 4 days, without oxygen for 4 minutes and without nerve supply for only 4 seconds.

This book reveals the secrets of using these four essential components of health to your advantage. Everyone knows they need these four things, but very few know how to really rev their body up with them. Knowledge is power, and this information will change your life!

A Quick Look at What's To Come

- *Food*—additives that destroy your health and longevity, the tricks of eating the right foods together, easily getting to the perfect pH balance, 5 pillars for harmonious aging and living
- *Water*—the secrets of the fountain of youth, illness and dehydration can be the same thing, how to get truly healthy drinking water
- *Oxygen*—the importance of breathing clean air, making your home safer and healthier with cleaner air, using hyperbaric oxygen chambers to treat and prevent disease
- *Nerve supply*—the best has been saved for last . . . the one thing that may be missing in your life that just may save your life

FOOD

From Fat to Fit: You Are What You Eat

One of the essentials for a healthy, disease-free life is a healthy diet. The nutrients found in food are the fuel that powers all of the body's activities; therefore, the right balance of foods is essential for the smooth running of the body. Choosing the right food helps the body grow and repair itself, provides protection from diseases and ultimately is responsible for maintaining optimum health, optimum energy levels and maximum lifespan.

Macro—and Micronutrients

Food is made up of a number of different types of nutrients. Carbohydrates, proteins and fats/oils are known as **macronutrients** because the body needs large quantities of them, while vitamins and minerals are considered **micronutrients** because they are needed in much smaller amounts.

- *Carbohydrates*—the body's major source of energy. Examples: rice, corn, potatoes, wheat.
- *Proteins*—provide the body with the raw materials needed for the growth and repair of cells, tissues and organs; can come from both animal and plant sources. Examples: meat, dairy, poultry, fish, beans, nuts.
- *Fats and Oils*—another source of energy; also provide the building blocks to construct cell membranes and help key systems in the body function properly. Examples: coconut oil, olive oil, butter, grape seed oil.
- *Vitamins*—needed in very small amounts for growth and for the body to function properly; some dissolve in water while others dissolve in fat. Examples: vitamin A, B vitamins, vitamin C, vitamin D, vitamin E, vitamin K.
- *Minerals*—chemical elements the body can't produce but are needed for optimal functioning of the body. Examples: calcium, magnesium, potassium, sodium, zinc and iodine.

When we talk about choosing a healthy diet, this really means two things:

1. Eating foods that benefit the body by providing both macro—and micro-nutrients
2. Eliminating foods that are harmful to your health

Unfortunately, even though most people know how important it is to eat healthy, only a few people do. But now, more and more people are turning from their old ways and joining the revolution of eating to live, rather than living to eat. If you haven't yet made that change it may be because you are short on time and energy, so you eat foods that are convenient rather than healthy. Or maybe you are accustomed to the taste of unhealthy foods, and prefer them to healthy foods. Eventually most people realize the importance of healthy eating when they get sick. But at this point it is often too late. The damage has already been done, but it is reversible if the steps in this book are followed.

Let's take a closer look at how the food you put in your body can affect your overall health.

Food Additives that Subtract from Your Health

Preservatives

For centuries, man has tried to keep his food fresh and edible for as long as possible. For example, in the old days, everyone from the Pilgrims to the pioneers preserved their meat with natural preservatives like salt. Today food manufacturers prevent bacterial and fungal growth with artificial food preservatives. These preservatives are claimed to be safe both by the manufacturers and the FDA, but the truth is that the abundance of artificial preservatives in our diet may lead to serious health problems.

Preservative	May Be Found In	Negative Effects
Sulfur dioxide, sulfites	Wines, dried fruits and vegetables	Hyperactivity, asthma attacks

Sodium nitrate, sodium nitrite	Bacon, ham, hotdogs, lunch meats, smoked fish, corned beef	Reduced blood transport of oxygen; cancer
Butylated hydroxyanisole (BHA)	Cereals, chewing gum, potato chips, vegetable oil, other oily foods	Cancer; high cholesterol; liver and kidney damage; infertility; immune system disorders; behavioral problems
Butylated hydroxytoluene (BHT) Note: banned in some countries	Potato flakes, dry breakfast cereals, enriched rice, foods containing animal fats and shortening	Tumors, cancer, cholesterol imbalances, hyperactivity, asthma attacks
Benzoic acid, sodium benzoate	Jam, jelly, juice, soft drinks, beer, margarine, pickled vegetables, barbecue sauce, condiments, salad dressings	Asthma attacks, rashes, eye irritation, hyperactivity, neurological problems; cancer

Label Lowdown: Some "natural" hot dogs and other processed/cured meats may boast "no added nitrite" but always be skeptical about this claim. While these products may not contain any added sodium nitrite, they are sometimes made with celery powder or celery juice, which are naturally high in nitrite. In fact, *The New York Times* reported that "natural" cured meats can have 10 times more nitrite than the conventionally cured meats.

Excitotoxins

Excitotoxins are substances that cause brain cells to become too excited. As a result, these cells start working so hard that eventually they die. Excitotoxins also affect the nervous system in other ways:

- Can alter brain development in fetuses, babies and young children
- Can destroy certain brain and nerve cells
- Can make cells produce too many hormones, altering our ability to remember/think, even in lower than toxic doses
- Stimulates production of harmful free radicals that damage tissues and cause aging and cancer
- Interferes with glucose entry into the brain, possibly leading to brain damage

Despite these major effects on brain development and function, most people have probably never heard of excitotoxins. As a result, these dangerous chemicals continue to be added in large concentrations to processed foods. Products especially high in excitotoxins include:

- Gravies
- Salad dressings (especially diet ones)
- Soups
- Diet foods and drinks
- Liquid amino acid preparations
- Anything that contains MSG or aspartame (NutraSweet)

Conditions Caused or Worsened
By Excitotoxins

- Brain damage
- Strokes
- AIDS dementia
- Migraine headaches
- Viral infections (Lyme disease, AIDS)
- Seizures
- Hepatic encephalopathy
- Degenerative brain disorders (Parkinson's, ALS, Alzheimer's)
- Immune suppression
- Episodic violence
- Learning disorders

Monosodium Glutamate (MSG)

The origins of MSG usage are found in the traditional Japanese practice of putting a type of seaweed in food to enhance its flavor. A chemical called glutamate found in the seaweed stimulates the cells in the tongue and brain, making foods taste better. As food producers began to package and can foods, they found that the flavor often lessened with time. For them, mono sodium glutamate (MSG) was the perfect solution, and by 1933, 10 million pounds of MSG were being produced and put into foods.

Food manufacturers assumed MSG was safe because it was derived from the amino acid glutamate that exists naturally in the body. It was even added to baby food without being tested! Then in 1957, two eye doctors conducted a study that showed that MSG totally destroyed all of the nerve cells in the retinal region of the eye of laboratory animals. Later, research conducted in the 1960s showed that not only did MSG kill eye cells but it killed critical parts of the brain as well, with a pattern of destruction that resembled the damage caused by strokes, severe low blood sugar and Alzheimer's.

This damage stems from the fact that the body doesn't know how to handle protein that has been chemically broken down into individual amino acids like glutamate. The body was designed to break down proteins slowly so amino acids don't flood the blood stream. When we eat MSG, our blood levels of glutamate can reach 20 times the normal levels and the brain, liver, muscles and the rest of our organs just aren't equipped to deal with concentrations like this.

> **Food for Thought:** Humans are more sensitive to the toxicity of MSG than any other animal. We are 5 times more sensitive than mice (the animals usually used in toxicity studies), and 20 times more sensitive than rhesus monkeys. Even more importantly, because their brains are still developing, newborns are 4 times more sensitive than adults!

Dangerous Health Effects of MSG

Studies in animals have confirmed that exposing babies to MSG can cause:

- Various organs, including the ovaries, testes, adrenal glands, kidneys, spleen and pituitary, to shrink to a significantly smaller size than normal
- Obesity that is very difficult to reduce with exercise or diet
- Abnormal reproductive function
- Impaired immune function
- Unprovoked rage, overt aggression and antisocial behavior
- Impaired heart and blood vessel function
- High triglycerides, cholesterol and VLDL levels, which are linked to a high risk of heart attack and stroke
- Altered hormonal control and responsiveness
- Disrupted intellectual development and difficulty learning
- Trouble concentrating or paying attention

And these effects can persist for the animal's entire life.

Hidden Sources of MSG

As more and more people have become aware of the dangers associated with MSG, the MSG manufacturers and the processed food industry have had to become sneakier about how they identify the MSG added to food. Therefore it is important to remember that MSG is a salt of glutamate. However, it isn't the sodium that is the issue; it's the glutamate that acts as an excitotoxin. As a result, it is vital to avoid all food additives that flood the body with glutamate, including hidden sources of MSG.

> **Label Lowdown:** Just because a package or a can states the food has "No MSG" or "No Added MSG" doesn't mean it is free of excitotoxins like glutamate. Some manufacturers use ingredient names on their labels that they think consumers won't recognize as MSG or glutamate. Also keep in mind that powerful excitotoxins like aspartate and L-cysteine are frequently added to foods and do not have to appear on the label according to current FDA rules.

Other names for MSG or glutamate:

- Glutamate
- Glutamic acid
- Monopotassium glutamate
- Calcium glutamate
- Natrium glutamate (natrium is Latin/German for sodium)
- Yeast extract, yeast food, yeast nutrient
- Autolyzed yeast, autolyzed yeast extract
- Torula yeast
- Autolyzed soy protein (or any protein that is "autolyzed")
- Hydrolyzed proteins, such as hydrolyzed vegetable protein, hydrolyzed plant protein, hydrolyzed whey protein, hydrolyzed pea protein, hydrolyzed corn protein, hydrolyzed corn gluten, hydrolyzed oat flour
- Calcium caseinate, sodium caseinate
- Textured protein, including Textured Vegetable Protein (TVP)

- Gelatin
- Soy protein, soy protein concentrate, soy protein isolate
- Soy milk
- Whey protein, whey protein concentrate, whey protein isolate
- Corn oil
- Kombu
- Miso

Food additives that *often* contain MSG or create MSG during processing:

- Carageenan
- Malt extract / flavoring
- Barley malt
- Maltodextrin
- Citric acid
- Soy sauce, soy sauce extract
- Bouillon, broth and stock
- Seasonings and/or spices (may contain between 30% to 60% MSG)
- Natural beef / chicken / pork flavoring
- Ultra-pasteurized milk powder and milk products
- Flavor(s) and flavoring(s) (may contain between 30% to 60% MSG)
- Natural flavor(s) and flavoring(s) (may contain between 30% to 60% MSG)
- Pectin
- Protease
- Fish sauce, fish sauce extract

MSG 'Red Flags' on Food Labels

- Glutamate
- Anything "hydrolyzed" (especially proteins)
- Anything "autolyzed"
- Anything "... protein"
- Anything "enzyme modified"
- Anything containing "enzymes"
- Anything "protein fortified"
- Anything "fermented"
- "Flavors" and/or "seasonings"

Aspartame

Aspartame is a chemical combination of two amino acids (phenylalanine and the excitotoxin aspartate) plus methanol. It was initially thought to be the perfect artificial sweetener because it is 150 times sweeter than an equal amount of sugar. As a result, aspartame (also known under the brand names Equal or NutraSweet) is currently used in:

- More than 5,000 food products, especially those claiming to be low calorie, diet or sugar free
- A number of medications, both prescription and over-the-counter
- Many beverages, including diet soft drinks and sugar-free drink mixes

However, aspartame is a powerful excitotoxin and accounts for approximately 70% of all complaints to the FDA. It has been linked to negative effects ranging from blindness to headaches to convulsions. This is because within 20 minutes at room temperature aspartame breaks down into several toxic and dangerous chemicals:

- *DKP (diketopiperazine),* which is converted in the body to a near duplicate of a powerful brain-tumor-causing agent
- *Formic acid* (ant venom)
- *Formaldehyde* (embalming fluid)
- *Methanol,* which is an extremely dangerous poison that causes blindness

Dangerous Health Effects of Aspartame

All kinds of physical and mental problems have been reported as a result of consuming aspartame, from DNA damage to cancer to hyperactivity, as well as dizziness and hallucinations. In 2005, researchers from the Ramazzini Foundation in Bologna, Italy, found that young rats fed aspartame at eight weeks old developed lymphomas and leukemias. In 2007, the same Italian researchers published a follow-up study that looked at exposing rats to aspartame *in utero.* This study found that this prenatal exposure to aspartame was enough to cause leukemias, lymphomas and breast cancer later in life.

> **Tip:** Everyone, especially young children and pregnant women, should avoid all foods and drinks that contain artificial sweeteners like aspartame (NutraSweet), saccharin (Sweet N Low, Equal), sucralose (Splenda) and acesulfame-K (Sweet One) due to their link to cancer. Instead, switch to products that contain all-natural sweeteners like Stevia

or xylitol and sweeten your foods with raw honey and blackstrap molasses.

Trans Fats: The Death of America

Trans fats are produced when liquid vegetable oils are chemically modified in a process, known as hydrogenation, hence their other name *partially hydrogenated oils*. This not only converts the oil into a semi-solid shortening (think Crisco or margarine), but also makes the oil less likely to spoil. As a result, food manufactures and restaurants like using trans fats because they:

- Help foods stay fresher for longer
- Have a longer shelf life
- Give foods a more desirable taste and texture
- Make foods less greasy
- Are cheap
- Can be used over and over again in commercial fryers

Foods Likely to Contain Trans Fats

- Fried fast foods like chicken, fish sandwiches and French fries
- Processed baked goods like crackers, cookies, cakes, donuts, muffins and pies
- Microwavable popcorn
- Canned biscuits
- Instant coffee beverages
- Shortenings and some margarines

Food for Thought: Since trans fat is often part of the oil restaurants use to fry food, a large serving of French fries can contain 5g of trans fat *or more*.

Dangerous Health Effects of Trans Fats

When it comes to your health, trans fat is considered by many experts to be the worst type of fat you can eat. In fact, an FDA committee concluded in 2004 that on a gram-for-gram basis, trans fat is even more harmful than the saturated fat most doctors warn about. This is because trans fat increases our risk of developing heart disease even more than the saturated fats found in butter, cheese and beef.

While saturated fats are known for their ability to raise total cholesterol levels, trans fat goes a step further by actually depleting your "good" (HDL) cholesterol as well. Since a combination of high LDL cholesterol and low HDL cholesterol is the most effective recipe for heart disease, trans fats really should be avoided at all costs.

The Shocking Truth About Cholesterol . . .

At a Glance

- Cholesterol is crucial for your body's production of hormones and for healthy cells
- Studies show that Lp(a), CRP, homocysteine, HbA1c and fibrinogen tests are better indicators of heart attack risk than total cholesterol and LDL

- The panel of nine "experts" who created the 2004 National Cholesterol Education Program guidelines were paid to lower the normal number for cholesterol, increasing the number of people taking statins from 13 million to 40 million
- Low cholesterol (below 156 mg/dL) can cause mood disorders, depression, aggression, violence and even suicide
- In studies with elderly people, **high** cholesterol was linked to a **longer** lifespan
- Folic acid, vitamins B6 and B12, and fish oil lower heart attack risk without the dangers of cholesterol-lowering medication

While doctors are generally most concerned about the way trans fats affect your cholesterol levels, trans fat has also been shown to have other harmful effects in the body:

- *Raises triglyceride levels*—triglycerides are a type of fat found in your blood. A high triglyceride level puts you at risk for developing hardening of the arteries (atherosclerosis) or thickening of the artery walls, which can lead to heart disease, diabetes, heart attack and stroke.
- *Increases Lp(a) lipoprotein*—Lp(a) is a type of LDL cholesterol found in your blood. When you eat foods that contain trans fat, the Lp(a) particles become smaller and denser, which encourages the buildup of dangerous plaques in your arteries.

- *Promotes inflammation*—inflammation is a natural process that helps your body deal with injury; however, it also may play a key role in the formation of fatty plaques in blood vessels. Consuming trans fat appears to damage the cells that line the blood vessels, which leads to inflammation. The tests CRP, homocysteine and HbA1c are good measures of your inflammation levels that everyone should have performed.

The toll trans fat takes on our heart health is tremendous. Researchers at the Harvard School of Public Health have estimated that trans fat causes about 50,000 premature deaths from heart attack every year. And, according to the Nurses' Health Study (the largest research study on women and long-term disease), trans fat intake doubles the risk of heart disease in women. It's no wonder that trans fats, aka partially hydrogenated oil, is considered one of the most harmful ingredients in our diets.

Food for Thought: When you eat a bag of potato chips, a plate of French fries or donut with your coffee it takes your body 51 days to breakdown and eliminate *half* of the hydrogenated fat you just consumed. In another 51 days, half of that (25%) is still in your body. 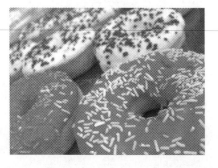 That means that after 102 days, *over 3 months*, you still haven't processed all of the trans fat you ate! Now think about all of the snacks, prepackaged and deep fried foods you eat every day and imagine how much trans fat is clogging up your body from years of eating this way.

Words to Live By: The Importance of Reading Labels

Just like with MSG, it's important to know the words to look for on food labels so you can figure out if the food contains trans fat. In this case, you need to look for the term "partially hydrogenated" vegetable oil, as it is the code name usually used for trans fat. However, just to make things even more confusing for the average consumer, "fully" or "completely" hydrogenated oil doesn't contain trans fat. This is because the process used to make fully or completely hydrogenated oil doesn't create trans-fats. Keep in mind though, if the label simply says "hydrogenated" vegetable oil, this could mean some trans fat is present.

Label Lowdown: Foods labeled "0g trans fat" are permitted by the FDA to contain half a gram (or less) trans fats per serving. This means you are still getting trans fats. "No trans fat," on the other hand, means none of these dangerous fats can be present at all.

How To Be a Smart Shopper

- Never go grocery shopping on an empty stomach because you will be more likely to make poor food choices and buy items on impulse. If you go shopping with your children, make sure to give them a satisfying snack before leaving home.

- Shop around the perimeter of the store. Most of the processed foods, which contain a lot of trans fats, preservatives and additives, are shelved in the inner aisles.

- Grab some quick meals, snacks and lunch items. By purchasing healthy foods that you can fix quickly at home (such as a stir-fry using fresh vegetables, or some raw nuts for a snack), you will be more likely to eat better even when you are in a hurry.

- Get in the habit of reading nutrition labels—the panel headed "Nutrition Facts." Make sure to look at all of the ingredients listed there, especially for words that disguise dangerous ingredients like MSG and trans fats.

- Finally, remember that you are ultimately responsible for the quality of food you have in your house. You and your family can only eat what is available. So shop wisely!

Finding the Perfect Match: The Power of Food Combining for Health And Weight Loss

It's not just what you eat that can make a difference in your health but how you eat it as well. The theory of "food combining" is based on the idea that you should only eat foods that are compatible with each other in terms of digestive chemistry. By only combining foods that have roughly the same digestion time, the body is able to digest and utilize the nutrients found in the meal to their full extent.

When you don't follow this advice, any quickly digested foods in your meal have to wait until the slowest foods to be digested leave the stomach—a process that can take 6 to 8 hours sometimes. During this holdup, foods like fruit, cooked and raw vegetables and some starches begin to decompose and ferment, which produces gas, acid and even alcohol. Talk about indigestion! Toxic particles produced by incomplete digestion can also pass into the bloodstream where they can cause allergic reactions or food sensitivities that manifest themselves as various health related problems like celiac disease, autism,

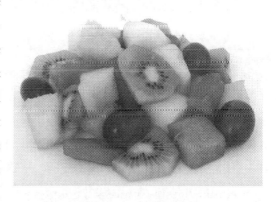

rheumatoid arthritis, type I diabetes and thyroid disease. Finally, undigested food particles left in the intestinal tract become food for unhealthy bacteria to feed upon, creating gas, bloating, a depleted immune system and more.

Understanding Digestive Chemistry:
When Opposites Don't Attract

Different foods require different digestive enzymes to completely break them down into nutrients the body can absorb and use. Some of these enzymes work best in an acidic environment while some need a non-acidic (alkaline) environment. Therefore anytime two or more foods are eaten at the same time that require opposite conditions for digestion, the digestive process is not optimal for at least one of the foods. This situation often leads to indigestion, bloating, gas, abdominal discomfort and poor absorption of nutrients.

> **Proteins** (meat, nuts, lentils, dairy) **require a highly acidic environment for digestion.**
>
> **Fats and carbohydrates** (grains, starchy vegetables, fruit and sugars) **require an alkaline environment for digestion.**

As a result, it is possible to eat large quantities of nutritious foods and get no benefit from them at all! For example, although cheese is rich in calcium, if we eat it with other foods that interfere with its proper digestion like bread, by the time the cheese reaches our small intestine, an alkaline digestive process is going on there, and very little (if any) of the calcium it contains will actually be absorbed. The calcium will make a chemical combination with the alkali and become non-absorbable. Therefore, it will pass through the intestinal tract and out of our body unused! This means that no matter how much cheese we eat, we may still suffer from calcium deficiency if the calcium is not absorbed.

Rule #1: Avoid mixing starchy foods with protein-rich foods at the same meal.

So instead of a ham sandwich for lunch that contains protein (ham) and starches (bread), eat a green salad with a chicken breast. Likewise, if you're having fats, don't eat any starches. If you're having bacon or eggs for breakfast, don't eat cereal or toast with it.

Food Combining Made Easy

- Instead of steak and potatoes, eat steak with asparagus or some other form of vegetable
- Instead of spaghetti and meatballs, eat spaghetti with steamed broccoli OR meatballs on a green salad
- Eat nuts as a snack by themselves rather than as a part of salads or other foods since they take hours to digest
- Fruits undergo no digestion in the stomach and are held up if eaten with anything else other than fruits; eat them 45 minutes or an hour away from a meal
- Forget the desserts—eaten on top of meals they are the last to leave the stomach, and therefore the sugar ferments causing gas and bloating

---

Rule #2: Chew each bite of food about 30 times or until is a thick paste rather than chunky. Remember, the stomach doesn't have any teeth!

Advocates of food combining also emphasize the importance of thoroughly chewing all food before swallowing. A researcher named

Abbe Spallanzani who made observations on gastric digestion in the 18th century, noted that when grapes and cherries were swallowed whole (even if they were completely ripe), they usually passed out of the body entirely unbroken. To further prove that the stomach was not very good at breaking things down, he swallowed some very thin wooden tubes that were designed so that the slightest pressure would crush them. Still, they passed through his digestive system completely unbroken. This confirms that we can only get nutritional value from those foods that enter our digestive system already crushed and chewed into almost a liquid.

Walking the Line: How to Maintain Acid-Alkaline Balance

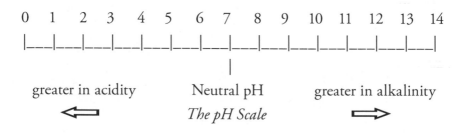

To be healthy our diet needs to include a balance of acidic and alkaline foods. Let's just take a minute here to refresh your memory about acids and bases. As you may (or may not) remember from high school chemistry class, a substance's acidity or alkalinity is measured according to its pH—or its potential (p) for freeing hydrogen (H) ions. The pH scale ranges from 0 to 14, with 7 indicating the ideal balance between acid and alkaline substances or a "neutral pH." Acids fall below neutral and range from 6 to 0, with 0 indicating a state of absolute acidity. Conversely, alkaline pHs fall above neutral and range from 8 to 14, with 14 corresponding to absolute alkalinity.

Most Americans Are Hopped Up on Acid

Our diet ultimately determines the acid-alkaline balance or imbalance in our bodies. In general, most Americans live on acid-forming, commercially-processed foods like beef, pork, pasta, hamburgers, hot dogs, frozen dinner, crackers, cookies, rice and dairy products. These foods create a lower, or more acidic, pH in the body. Also, while we are filling up on health-robbing, acid-forming foods, we are also avoiding health-promoting, alkaline-forming foods such as fruits, vegetables, whole grains, beans and other foods high in fiber. As a result, the real problem is an alkaline deficiency rather than consuming too much acid. This way of eating spells disaster for our health.

> **Food for Thought:** Most Americans—68 to 91%—don't eat the recommended amount of fruits and vegetables every day. Fruits and vegetables should make up half of our daily food intake!

A Quick Guide to Acidic and Alkaline Foods	
Acid-Producing Foods:	*Alkaline-Producing Foods:*
• Spaghetti	• Apricots
• Corn flakes	• Kiwis
• White rice	• Cherries
• Rye bread	• Bananas
• White bread	• Strawberries
• Whole milk	• Peaches
• Lentils	• Oranges
• Beef	• Lemon juice
• Pork	• Pears

Very Acid-Producing Foods:

- Parmesan cheese
- Soft cheeses
- Hard cheeses
- Gouda cheese
- Cottage cheese
- Brown rice
- Rolled oats
- Whole-wheat bread
- Peanuts
- Walnuts
- Salami/lunch meat
- Liver sausage
- Chicken
- Cod
- Herring
- Trout
- Eggs

- Pineapple
- Apples
- Watermelon
- Celery
- Carrots
- Zucchini
- Broccoli/cauliflower
- Green peppers
- Cucumbers
- Tomatoes
- Eggplant
- Lettuce
- Green beans
- Onions
- Mushrooms
- Mineral water

Very Alkaline-Producing Foods:

- Spinach
- Raisins
- Dates

* Note: All fruits and vegetables are alkaline producing unless they have been pickled or marinated. Therefore, I strongly suggest having a greens drink, such as Green Vibrance, everyday. The high concentration of alkalizing ingredients, such as green veggies, edible grasses and beneficial green algae, will help to bring your body into pH balance. I drink greens daily.

Too Much Acid Erodes Our Health and Well Being

The body generally functions at its best when its overall pH is neutral or slightly alkaline. The normal range for this optimum pH is very narrow, between 7.36 and 7.42. If the pH of the body is thrown off in either direction (usually by the diet), the body functions less efficiently and illness and death can result.

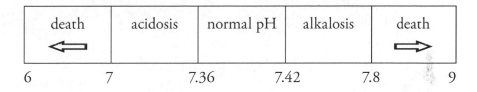

Fatal acidosis to fatal alkalosis

Because of our typical acid-forming diet, most people's pH falls in the acid range of 6.2 to 6.4. Just this slight lean toward the acidic end of the spectrum forces the body to borrow essential minerals like calcium, sodium, potassium and magnesium from vital organs and bones to neutralize the acid and safely remove it from the body. Because of this strain, the body can suffer severe and prolonged damage due to high acidity—a condition that may go undetected for years.

Just as too much acid can eat away at your car battery, acid overload promotes:

- Osteoporosis—weak, brittle bones, hip fractures and bone spurs
- Weak muscles
- Eroded cartilage

- Stiffness and achiness in the morning
- Brain, heart and blood vessel damage
- Diabetes
- High blood pressure
- Weight gain and obesity
- Bladder and kidney conditions, including kidney stones
- Immune deficiency
- Yeast overgrowth
- Bacterial and viral infections
- Cancer
- Low energy levels and chronic fatigue
- Poor circulation
- Sexual problems
- Sleep issues
- Joint pain and leg cramps at night
- Premature wrinkling and other aging issues

The 5 Pillars Of Supplementation For Harmonious Living

A final important aspect to achieving health through food is preventing deficiencies. There are literally thousands of supplements on the market that claim they will help boost your health and prevent disease, but which ones will provide you with actual benefits?

There are five different classes or 'pillars' of supplementation that will help you on the path toward harmonious living:

1. *Whole Food Multivitamin*—Taking a multivitamin is a great way to top up the vitamins and minerals that are missing in your diet. Unfortunately, not all multivitamins use materials taken from natural sources like plants, fruits and vegetables. Instead, many commercially produced multivitamins use synthetic versions of real vitamins that are produced in the lab. These are the same types of "vitamins" that are used as additives in processed foods. Because they are not natural, your body only absorbs a small percentage and is able to utilize even less. So what do I recommend? A whole food-based multivitamin that has very little to no additional ingredients and no iron.

    WARNING: Be very careful purchasing your supplements from large commercial chain stores. It is always best to buy from local health food stores.

2. *Fish Oil*—Since the typical American diet generally contains too many omega-6 and—9 fatty acids, most of us do not get enough of two important nutrients: DHA and EPA. Multiple studies have shown that taking a fish oil supplement can lower your triglyceride level; reduce your risk of having a heart attack, dangerous abnormal heart rhythm or stroke; slow the buildup

of fatty plaques in your arteries; prevent hardening of the arteries; lower your blood pressure; prevent neurodegenerative diseases like Alzheimer's; help improve children's IQs; and contribute to the healthy development of fetuses when taken by pregnant women. Look for a fish oil supplement with 750 mg DHA and 1100 mg EPA. Adults can take double this dose, while children should take half the recommended dose. Do not take fish oil if you are on blood thinning medication without first asking your doctor if it is okay.

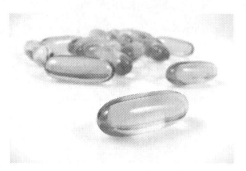

3. *Antioxidant Complex*—Antioxidants neutralize damage-causing free radicals in the body. While free radicals are produced during normal bodily functions, they can damage cellular DNA, increase the stickiness of cholesterol and promote aging when present in high quantities. As a result, antioxidant supplements may help protect against cancer, degenerative eye diseases such as age-related macular degeneration and glaucoma, Alzheimer's and other degenerative brain diseases, heart attack and stroke, as well as strengthen the immune system. Good ingredients to look for in an antioxidant supplement are vitamins C and E, coenzyme Q10, selenium, alpha lipoic acid (ALA) and N-acetyl cysteine.

4. *Probiotics*—These friendly bacteria help boost the number of health-promoting microorganisms that live in your gut. This is important because these "good" bacteria are responsible for the proper functioning of your immune system; for protecting

against disease-causing microorganisms that may want to live in your gut; and for aiding in the complete digestion and absorption of food and nutrients. Probiotic supplements have been used to treat diarrhea, Crohn's disease, irritable bowel syndrome, urinary tract infections, eczema, respiratory tract infections and much more.

Probiotics are also essential for those of you who have taken antibiotics. Antibiotics kill off all of the good bacteria in your gut, compromising your immune system. Therefore, without probiotic supplementation, you may be running back to the doctor frequently for infections of some sort. Save yourself the time and money and take probiotics on a daily basis.

5. *Digestive Enzymes*—A diet that consists mainly of cooked food requires the pancreas to work overtime producing enzymes. As we age, all of this extra effort adds up, leaving the pancreas exhausted. By taking a digestive enzyme supplement with meals, we can help the body digest foods, improving the breakdown of foods and increasing the amount of nutrients our bodies absorb. This prevents gas and bloating. Also, when taken on an empty stomach these enzymes help reduce damaging inflammation throughout the body, reducing any stiffness and achiness you may feel.

BONUS: My personal morning favorite is a *greens drink in the morning*. It helps decrease acid in the body, leading to a faster metabolism, weight loss, better digestion, surcharged energy, less stiffness and achiness and faster recovery time.

WATER

Secrets Of The Fountain Of Youth Revealed

Water is the basis of life. Water not only makes up 60 to 70% of our body weight, but also serves a range of purposes. Water is essential for removing wastes, maintaining a healthy metabolism and controlling our body temperature, heart rate and blood pressure. It's no wonder then that our bodies function and feel better when they have a healthy supply of water.

> **Did You Know:** Your blood is 83% water, your brain is 74% water, your muscles are 75% water and even your bones are 22% water.

Water, Water Everywhere Yet Not Enough We Drink

Drinking enough water seems like such a simple thing to do yet 75% of Americans are always dehydrated. This is because we lose 1-2 liters of water a day just by breathing! Exercising, sweating, diarrhea, hot temperature and high altitudes can increase the amount of water we lose even more.

Because we lose so much fluid through our sweat, urine, exhaled air and bowel movements, it has to be replaced throughout the day to keep our body functioning normally. However, this is where the problem lies. Most people wait until they feel thirsty before drinking water, but having a dry feeling in your mouth means that your body has been already dehydrated for quite some time. This is because thirst does not develop until your body fluids are depleted well below the levels required to keep your body functioning at optimum levels. Therefore a dry mouth or thirst should be considered the last outward sign of dehydration, not your first signal to get a glass of water.

> **Did You Know:** Typically when you feel hungry, this is a sign that you are dehydrated.

Dehydration: An Underlying Cause of Damage, Illness and Premature Aging

So what happens when your body becomes dehydrated? Picture your body as a juicy plum that has just been picked from the tree. Without water, dehydration sets in and the interior of the plum begins to shrivel and its skin begins to wrinkle, eventually causing the plum to become a prune. This is exactly what happens to your body. Water loss causes both internal and external structures to change, leaving your internal cells damaged and your skin looking old and tired.

Common Physical Signs of Dehydration	General Feelings that Accompany Dehydration
• Dry, sticky mouth • Excessive thirst • Infrequent or dark urination • Muscle weakness or cramping • Headache • Rapid heartbeat and/or breathing • Dizziness or lightheadedness • Not sleeping well • Sunken eyes • Few or no tears when crying • Lack of sweating • Dry skin • Constipation	• Tiredness • Irritability • Confusion • Anxiety • Depression • Feeling flushed • Feeling dejected • Feeling heavy-handed • Having irresistible cravings • Being afraid of crowds or leaving the house

While these are the classic symptoms that doctors look for in cases of dehydration, dehydration doesn't affect everyone in the same way. Your body is made up of trillions of cells so dehydration can settle in to any area of your body and produce very different signals as a result. Unfortunately, most of these indicators of dehydration are not understood by the medical community and are treated instead as symptoms of many of the most common diseases and conditions affecting Americans today.

High Blood Pressure

Another common indicator of gradually occurring dehydration is a steady increase in blood pressure. Your blood vessels have been designed to handle repeated fluctuations in blood volume. Each of your blood vessels is built like a flexible tube, with a central passage (lumen) that is able to open and close depending on the amount of blood that is inside it. When you are dehydrated, the amount of blood in your vessels decreases. Your body immediately responds by shutting down the tiniest 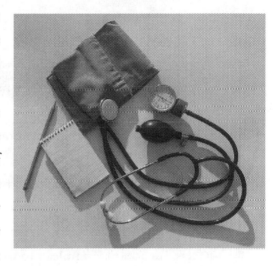 blood vessels known as capillaries, and eventually your larger vessels tighten their walls (creating a smaller lumen space) in order to keep the blood vessels full.

This tightening causes the pressure to rise in the arteries, a condition known as hypertension or high blood pressure. While high blood pressure can cause serious health problems, the result of not reducing the space in the blood vessels would be more disastrous. If the blood vessels did not decrease their lumen size, gases would separate from the blood and fill up the extra space, causing gas locks that would kill us.

Unfortunately, most mainstream healthcare professionals don't realize that hypertension and another condition that you will learn about in the next section are a response to dehydration in the body. As a result, they prescribe diuretics to remove water through urination and lower blood pressure, but that further dehydrates the body. In time, this can cause plaques to develop in the arteries that feed the heart and brain, leading to heart attacks and small or massive strokes. Such treatment can also cause kidney disease. Doesn't drinking enough water sound like a better and safer alternative?

Other Painful Conditions

According to Dr. Batmanghelidj, water is also important for preventing and curing a long list of other painful conditions:

- *Heartburn* is a sign of dehydration in the upper part of the gastrointestinal (GI) tract and is a major thirst signal from your body. If you take antacids or other heartburn medications to treat this pain it may go away temporarily, but it will not resolve the underlying dehydration. In time, allowing this water shortage to continue can lead to inflammation of the stomach and duodenum, hiatal hernia, ulceration and eventually cancer of the liver, pancreas and other gastrointestinal organs.
- *Arthritis* is a sign of dehydration in the affected joint. Water is one of the most important components of the fluid that cushions your joints. Without it your bones can rub together, causing chronic pain and serious damage to the joint. Therefore, increasing your water intake will help rebuild this fluid and alleviate the problem without exposing you to the additional damage that pain medications can cause.
- *Low back pain* is often caused by a water shortage in your spine. Just like in your joints, there are water cushions between your spinal vertebrae (called discs) that support the weight of the body. Increasing your water intake will help replenish this fluid

and nourish cartilage cells, reducing pain and preventing future deformity.

- *Chest pain (angina)* is caused by dehydration in the heart and lungs. It can be treated with increased water intake under a doctor's supervision.

- *Constipation* and *colitis* is often caused by dehydration in the large intestine. These conditions are linked because water is essential to lubricate the passage of feces. It is important to drink enough water because persistent constipation can lead to fecal impacting, diverticulitis, hemorrhoids and polyps later in life. It can also greatly increase your risk of developing colorectal cancer by extending the amount of time the cells that line your intestine are in contact with harmful wastes.

---

25 Reasons To Stay Well Hydrated

1. Without water, nothing can live.
2. Water generates electrical and magnetic energy inside our cells, giving our bodies the power to live.
3. Water helps prevent the DNA damage that can lead to cancer and makes it easier for the body to fix any damage that has already occurred.
4. Water boosts the immune system, making it more effective and efficient at protecting our bodies from harmful infections and cancer cells.
5. Water is essential for breaking down food into smaller pieces. It also plays a major role in the absorption and metabolism of essential nutrients, vitamins and minerals.

6. Water increases how fast the body can absorb essential nutrients from food and helps transport all substances around the body.

7. Water increases how efficiently red blood cells can collect oxygen from the lungs.

8. Water brings cells oxygen and takes waste gases to the lungs for disposal.

9. Water clears toxic wastes from different parts of the body, taking them to the liver and kidneys for removal.

10. Water is the main lubricant in the joints and helps prevent arthritis and back pain.

11. Water helps form shock-absorbing cushions in the spinal discs.

12. Water is the best lubricating laxative and prevents constipation.

13. Water dilutes the blood to the ideal concentration so that it flows freely and prevents solids from settling in the blood.

14. Water keeps the arteries to the heart and brain from becoming clogged, reducing the risk of heart attacks and strokes. A study reported that people who drink more than five glasses of water a day were less likely to die from a heart attack or heart disease than those who drank fewer than two glasses a day.

15. Water is essential for the body's cooling and warming systems.

16. Water is needed for the brain to produce all of its chemical signals and hormones.

17. Water helps reduce stress, anxiety and depression.

18. Water restores normal sleep patterns and helps reduce fatigue.

19. Water makes the skin smoother and helps reduce signs of aging.

20. Water gives luster and shine to the eyes and helps prevent glaucoma.

21. Water helps remove toxins from the body, protecting against bladder cancer. The risk of bladder cancer decreases by about 7% for every 8-ounce increase of daily fluid intake.

22. Water decreases premenstrual pains and hot flashes.

23. Water helps sex hormone production, thereby reducing impotence and increasing libido.

24. Water clears toxic sediments that may have been deposited in the tissue spaces, joints, kidneys, liver, brain and skin.

25. The human body has no stored water reserves that it can use during periods of dehydration. So you must drink regularly throughout the day!

Fill 'er Up: How to Stay Hydrated

Now that you know how important drinking enough water is, you are probably wondering just how much water you should be getting every day. Many people follow what's known as the 8 by 8 rule—drinking eight 8-ounce glasses of water per day (which equals about 2 quarts or 1.8 liters). However, the exact amount of water you need isn't so cut and dry. It varies based on your body weight, activity level and climate.

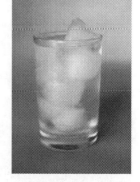

A really good way to figure out how much water you should be drinking is to divide your weight (in pounds) by two. The number you get is the amount of water (in ounces) that you need each day. For example, if you weigh 200 pounds, you should drink 100 ounces (3.13 quarts, 2.98 liters or about 10-12 cups) of water a day. But if you weigh 130 lbs, you should be drinking 65 ounces of water a day (about eight 8-ounce servings).

After that, you can look at your urine and urination patterns to see if the amount of water you are drinking is actually optimal for your body. When you are drinking enough, you will be urinating every two to four hours and your urine will be almost clear in color.

Monitoring Your Urine

A hydrated body produces *clear, colorless* urine.
A somewhat dehydrated body produces *yellow* urine.
A severely dehydrated body produces *orange or dark-colored* urine.

It is also important to realize that your body can only absorb about 4 ounces of water every 10 minutes. Therefore, it is important to be proactive with your drinking habits—aim to drink one glass of pure water every hour you are awake. For many people this may seem like a daunting task, especially if they believe they don't like the taste of water or that it is boring to drink. However, there are a number of things you can do to make getting enough water every day a little easier:

- Start and finish your day with a glass of water. Morning is when you are most full of toxins and dehydrated so a glass of water will help start your morning right. This will also help reduce constipation.

- Take regular water breaks throughout the day.
- Carry a stainless steel water bottle with you during work hours and when you are away from home for long periods of time.
- Avoid caffeinated and sugary drinks as much as possible. Caffeine is a diuretic and dehydrates. Also, the sugars in drinks like fruit juices can slow your body's ability to absorb fluids.
- Drink water before and after eating. Try to drink a glass of water half an hour before eating and half an hour after eating to help the digestive process. If you drink water while you eat, it dilutes the digestive juices, slowing digestion.
- Drink something before, during and after you exercise, especially if it is hot. You can lose up to 2 liters of fluid per hour while exercising, so drink water every 15-20 minutes during your workout.
- Keep a glass or stainless steel bottle of water next to your bed
- Eat more water-rich foods like watermelon, which is 92% water, tomato that is 95% water and egg that is about 74% water.
- Add fresh mint leaves, slices of strawberry, apple, lemon or lime to your water to keep your taste buds interested. Always keep a pitcher of "fruit water" in the refrigerator so you have great-tasting water available immediately.
- Drink hot or cold herbal teas—green tea, chai, chamomile, mint, raspberry leaf or cinnamon/apple, but be aware of the amount of sugar added. You will also want to avoid drinks made with artificial sweeteners.
- Always remember to drink before you get thirsty.

More than Meets the Eye: Finding Pure, Clean Drinking Water is Harder than It Looks

Our health is dependent not only on the quantity of the water we drink, but also the quality. Natural pure water is the best choice, but how do you know what natural pure water is when there are so many possible water-related products and sources of water?

'Fresh from Mountain Streams' and Other Myths of Bottled Water

Americans now drink more bottled water than any other country, mainly because we see it as a healthier alternative to tap water. However, bottled water is not necessarily any safer than tap water. In fact, it is often nothing more than tap water that may or may not have been filtered, according to a scientific study conducted by the Natural Resources Defense Council (NRDC).

The NRDC study tested more than 1,000 bottles of 103 different brands of bottled water. While most of the water was found to be of high quality, some brands were contaminated. Approximately one-third of the bottled waters tested contained potentially harmful synthetic organic chemicals and/or bacteria. Plus there was arsenic in at least one sample at levels that exceeded the allowable limits found in either state or bottled water industry standards or guidelines.

This is potentially due to a lack of regulation and oversight. The Food and Drug Administration (FDA) is meant to be the federal agency responsible for bottled water safety; however, according to FDA rules, 60-70% of bottled water sold in the US are completely exempt from federal regulations because they are packaged and sold within the same state. And, to make matters worse, roughly one out of five states don't regulate these waters either!

But even falling within the FDA's purview doesn't necessarily make bottled water any purer. In fact, city tap water has to be tested more frequently for bacterial and chemical contaminants than bottled water. In addition, the rules for bottled water allow for some contamination by E. coli or fecal coliform (which indicates possible contamination with fecal matter), while tap water rules completely prohibit any confirmed contamination with these bacteria. Similarly, there are no requirements for bottled water to be disinfected or tested for parasites such as cryptosporidium or giardia, unlike the rules for big city tap water systems that use surface water sources.

The companies that market bottled waters push the image that their water comes from pristine, pure sources. However, in many cases this isn't true at all. For example, the NRDC observed:

- A brand of "Spring Water" showed a picture of a lake surrounded by mountains on the label. However, the water was actually taken from an industrial parking lot next to a hazardous waste site.
- Before FDA intervention, Alasika™ bottled water claimed to be "Alaska Premium Glacier Drinking Water: Pure Glacier Water From the Last Unpolluted Frontier, Bacteria Free" on their label, despite being taken from a public water supply.

Did You Know: Almost all bottled water is acidic with a pH ranging from 4-6.

The Perils of Plastic

It's not just the water that may be suspect, but also the plastic bottles they come in. Plastic is not the harmless compound that most of us think it is. Toxic chemicals like Bisphenol A (BPA) have been shown to leach out of both single-use and reusable plastic water bottles into the water to be absorbed by our bodies. In fact, a recent survey by the Centers for Disease Control established that virtually all Americans (more than 90%) have detectable levels of BPA in their bodies. This is quite scary because BPA has a chemical structure similar to the hormone estrogen. When it gets in our bodies, it can set off a chain reaction of estrogen responses in the male and female body and upset the natural balance of hormonal messages, even at very low doses.

More than a hundred scientific studies have shown that BPA is linked to a wide range of negative health effects, including:

- Breast cancer
- Prostate cancer
- Uterine cancer
- Early puberty
- Reduced sperm count
- Insulin resistance and type II diabetes
- Miscarriage
- Downs Syndrome
- Changes in brain chemistry and behavior, including hyperactivity, increased aggressiveness, changes in response to fear-provoking or painful stimuli, impaired learning, altered sexual behavior and increased susceptibility to addiction
- Obesity in adults due to *in utero* exposure
- Impaired immune function

- Decreased anti-oxidant enzyme levels, which leaves your body at risk for accumulating cellular and DNA damage

Despite the abundance of scientific studies that clearly link BPA to hormonal, developmental and other abnormalities in both animals and humans, the FDA issued a statement on August 15, 2008 reaffirming the safety of products containing low levels of BPA. However, nothing was said about the effects of repeated exposure to BPA over many years or the effect hormones can have on BPA in our bodies.

Because of the health risks associated with plastic, it is best to use a stainless steel water bottle to help you stay hydrated. Stainless steel water bottles are 100% recyclable, durable, do not alter the taste of its contents and are almost as lightweight as plastic. Most importantly though, stainless steel water bottles are free from toxic chemicals like BPA and are even safe to use with hot liquids.

A Little Spring Cleaning: Filtering Your Tap Water

Our drinking water from the tap starts out filled with dangerous contaminants like nitrate, arsenic, microorganisms, pharmaceuticals and chemicals from pesticide runoff, but many of these contaminants are removed once this water reaches a municipal treatment plant. Still, by the time it reaches our taps, there can still be at least 315 pollutants, according to an Environmental Working Group drinking water quality analysis of almost 20 million records obtained from state water officials. Therefore, good water filters offer a last line of defense between our bodies and these toxins that can cause harmful health effects, like cancer.

Arsenic

Arsenic is a natural element found in the earth's crust. It is used in industry and agriculture, as well as being a byproduct of copper smelting, mining and coal burning. It is also a deadly poison that has infiltrated our water supply. Based on the results of a NRDC report conducted in February 2000, as many as 56 million people in the 25 states included in the research were drinking water that contained unsafe levels of arsenic. This can lead to bladder, lung and skin cancer, and may cause kidney and liver cancer as well. A 1999 study published by the National Academy of Science also found that arsenic:

- Damages the central and peripheral nervous systems
- Harms the heart and blood vessels
- Causes serious skin problems
- May cause birth defects and reproductive problems

Chlorine

Surprisingly, one of the most dangerous contaminants to our health is actually added to drinking water as a part of the treatment process. Chlorine, which is added as an inexpensive disinfectant to drinking water, is also a known poison to the body. It is certainly not a coincidence that chlorine gas was used as a deadly weapon during World War I. When inhaled, this gas can severely burn the lungs and other body tissues, and it is no less powerful when it is drank in water. In fact, the US Council of Environmental Quality recently released a report showing that the risk of cancer is 93% higher in people who drink chlorinated water than those who did not.

Think About It: Every time we drink unfiltered tap water, we are essentially drinking water with bleach in it!

Chlorine in drinking water has been linked to at least three different types of cancer:

- *Bladder and Rectal Cancer*—Chlorine interacts with organic compounds found in water to create trihalomethanes (THMs). When THMs enter the body, they accelerate the production of free radicals, which go on to damage or destroy vital cells in the body and can lead to cancer. Because so much of the water we drink eventually ends up in our bladder and/or rectum, drinking THMs in our water is particularly damaging to these organs.
- *Breast Cancer*—Recent research has found that chlorine compounds can buildup in breast tissue. In fact, researchers discovered that women with breast cancer have 50-60% higher levels of organochlorines (chlorine byproducts) in their breast tissue than women without breast cancer.

Water filters are one of the only water purification methods that are capable of removing chlorine and other cancer-causing chemicals from tap water. In its May 17, 2010 report, the President's Cancer Panel recommended that people use home filtering devices to decrease their exposure to cancer-causing and hormone-disrupting chemicals. Of course, check to make sure that the water filter you choose is proven to be able to remove all these toxic contaminants like arsenic and chlorine, plus potentially harmful bacteria.

Understanding Different Types of Water

- *Mineral Water*—Mineral water usually comes from a natural well or spring and must contain a specific quantity of minerals. These minerals, like calcium and magnesium, are good for your overall health.
- *Distilled Water*—Distilled water is produced by boiling water to create vapor. This vapor is then collected and cooled until it becomes a liquid again. Because solid materials within the water are too heavy to be carried by the vapor, the water that is produced is completely free of minerals as well as contaminants. However, I do not recommend drinking distilled water because it has a tendency to pull minerals out of the bloodstream and other cells and tissues.
- *Purified Water*—Purified water is produced when contaminants and/or minerals are removed from any water source (tap water, well water, etc.) using a filter or ionizer.

The Best Solution: Ionized and Alkaline Water

Another way to improve your health and water is to alkalize or ionize it using a special machine. Alkaline water machines are not the same thing as water purifiers. Instead of simply filtering out the harmful elements in tap water, alkaline water machines fundamentally alter the water to make it healthier for your body. But it is important to first filter the water before alkalizing it!

Firstly, ionized alkaline water has a pH between 7 and 10. If you think back to the previous section, decreasing the acidity of your body has numerous health benefits. Also, alkaline water looks different under a microscope. Normal water molecules usually form clusters of about 13 molecules or more. However, after being ionized, alkaline water clusters are much smaller, generally with just 6 molecules in a cluster. Although it may not sound like much, this difference is very important. It helps the body use water clusters more efficiently and hydrates your body more effectively.

Other health benefits of alkaline water include:

- Increased clarity and energy
- Weight loss
- Symptom improvement for chronic diseases, including diabetes, arthritis and other inflammatory diseases
- Protects cell DNA from damage caused by free radicals
- Prevents cancer growth and spread
- Reduces bone weakening and prevents osteoporosis
- Prevents diabetes
- Anti-aging effects

OXYGEN

A Breath of Fresh Air: The Most Vital Element for Our Health

Our bodies are designed to run on oxygen, and every day we take at least 17,000 breaths to ensure that we have enough of this precious gas to remain healthy. As we breathe in, our lungs absorb oxygen and pass it into our bloodstream so it can be distributed throughout our bodies to help nourish every single cell in our system.

Think About It: While we need (on average) about two quarts of clean water every day, our bodies require approximately 15,000 quarts of air.

Essential Roles of Oxygen in the Body

- Oxidizes or "burns" food to create energy and heat for our bodies
- Used by the mitochondria found in all of our cells to generate chemical energy

> - Oxidizes or "burns" waste materials that would otherwise poison our cells
> - Serves as a component of many of the molecules that make up our body tissues

The earth contains about 6,000 billion tons of air, roughly 20% of which is oxygen, so quantity-wise, we're good to go. Unfortunately, the quality of the air we breathe is another story. So if you are serious about becoming and staying healthy, it's time to think about what you are breathing in besides oxygen.

Don't Let Your Health Go Up in Smoke: The Importance of Breathing Clean Air

While you can't choose when and where you breathe, you can make some decisions on the quality of the air you breathe. This has a huge impact on our health. In fact, research has shown that the cleaner the air you breathe, the longer you will live. In 2009, researchers from the Harvard School of Public Health compared the average lifespan of people living in 51 U.S. cities with varying levels of air pollution. During the roughly 20 years studied, reductions in concentrations of fine particles—those most hazardous to human health—had a beneficial effect on residents' health, adding five months to their average lifespan. In the cities with the largest improvements in air quality, this increase in lifespan jumped to 10 months.

Air Pollutants That Negatively Impact Health

- *Airborne Particles*—a complex mixture of solid and liquid particles that are suspended in the air. The major components are sulfate, nitrates, ammonia, sodium chloride, carbon, mineral dust and water.

- *Ozone (O_3)*—three atoms of oxygen linked together in a very energetic combination. It is formed when sunlight reacts with pollutants from car and industry emissions and is a major component of smog. When inhaled, ozone can damage sensitive tissues in the upper and lower respiratory tract.

- *Nitrogen Dioxide (NO_2)*—a brownish gas that mostly comes from power plants and cars. It reacts with other types of pollution in the air to form even more harmful chemicals. When inhaled, nitrogen dioxide causes lung irritation, inflammation and a suppressed immune system. As a result, children exposed to high levels of nitrogen dioxide have been shown to have an increased risk of developing respiratory infections.

- *Carbon Monoxide (CO)*—a colorless, odorless gas produced when fuels are burned. Once inhaled, carbon monoxide reacts with hemoglobin in the blood, preventing the uptake and transport of oxygen and decreasing the amount of oxygen delivered to vital organs like the heart and the brain.

- *Sulfur Dioxide (SO_2)*—a colorless gas with a sharp odor that is produced by burning coal, oil and diesel fuel. If inhaled, most sulfur dioxide is absorbed in the upper respiratory tract and does not reach the lung's airways. However, even the small amounts that do penetrate the airways can trigger illness and death, especially in people with asthma.

Breathing in harmful particles like dust, smog, soot, smoke and other poisonous gases can have serious short—and long-term effects on our health. In the short term, air pollution can aggravate conditions like asthma and emphysema, often with horrible consequences. During the infamous 1952 "Smog Disaster" in London, 4,000 people died in the span of a few days because of inhaling high concentrations of pollution. Years of breathing in tiny particles smaller than a human hair is known to increase illness and death rates from lung cancer, chronic obstructive pulmonary disease (COPD) and emphysema.

> **Did You Know?** Chronic exposure to particles, sulfur dioxide and nitrogen dioxide have been shown to increase nonspecific chronic respiratory symptoms by up to 300%!

In addition to damaging the lungs, air pollution poses a threat to cardiovascular health as well. A study published in the *Journal of the American Medical Association* in 2002 reported that when air pollution levels suddenly increase, not only is there an increase in deaths from asthma, pneumonia and emphysema, but there is also an increase in the number of deaths from heart attacks and strokes. A separate study published in the journal *Epidemiology* demonstrated that for every increase in fine particles by 10 micrograms per cubic meter, heart-disease-related deaths rose by 25%.

Even relatively low concentrations of air pollutants are related to negative health effects:

- Respiratory infections
- Lung cancer

- Asthma
- Chronic bronchitis
- Aggravation of emphysema
- Headaches
- Heart disease
- Leukemia
- Irritation of eyes, ears, nose, throat, lungs, and sinuses
- Nausea
- Dizziness
- Fatigue
- Drowsiness
- Allergic reactions
- Persistent cough
- Insomnia
- Joint and muscle pain
- Mental confusion
- Memory loss
- Depression
- Damage to the brain, nerves, liver or kidneys

Children are particularly vulnerable to the negative effects of air pollution. Part of this is because, relative to their size, children inhale more deeply and trap more airborne particles and pollutants in their lungs than both adolescents and adults. Children also have higher metabolisms than adults; they take in 20% to 50% more air than adults, and spend more time outdoors than adults, which further increases their susceptibility to pollution-related health problems.

A study conducted in The Netherlands investigated the relationship between traffic-related air pollution (nitrogen dioxide, fine particles and soot) and childhood development of asthma and other respiratory diseases and infections. By the age of 2, children who were exposed to higher levels of air pollution were more likely to suffer from wheezing, physician-diagnosed asthma, ear/nose/throat infections, and flu/serious

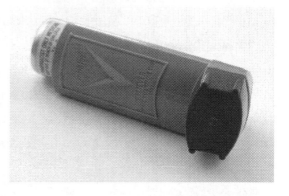

colds. And air pollution only makes things worse once respiratory complications develop. Based on the results of the Children's Health Study, children diagnosed with asthma experience more asthma symptoms when they live in neighborhoods with higher levels of air pollution and participate in three or more competitive sports.

An Inside Job: The Threat of Indoor Air Pollution to Your Health

While two-thirds of people in the United States live in areas with air that the Environmental Protection Agency (EPA) considers unhealthy, staying inside isn't exactly a better solution. The typical level of indoor pollutants can be 25 to 100 times higher than outdoor levels, even in our biggest cities. This is a huge problem, especially since the average American adult spends about 90% of their time indoors.

> **Did You Know?** Indoor air quality is one of the EPA's top five environmental risks to public health.

But where does all of this pollution come from? Two words—toxic chemicals. The average American home contains a combined total of at least 63,000 different chemicals, and every day at least 1,000 new ones are invented. While many of these chemicals are toxic, they often become even more so when they interact with each other inside a closed environment. In addition to the pollutants caused by household cleaners, smoke, exhaust and other things, the air inside your house can contain up to 30 million particles of dust per cubic foot!

Think About It: A baby crawling on the floor inhales the equivalent of 4 cigarettes a day due to the gases from carpets, molds, mildews, fungi, dust mites, etc. A better option are hardwood and bamboo flooring.

Major Sources of Indoor Air Pollution

- *Formaldehyde*—a toxic chemical commonly used as a bonding agent and preservative in building products and household goods. Examples: plywood, particle board, paneling, cabinets, furniture, countertops, curtains, carpets, upholstery fabrics, linens, insulation, shampoos, makeup, toothpastes, perfumes, hairsprays, soaps, toilet tissue, milk cartons, car bodies and household cleaners. Formaldehyde is considered to be harmful to human health and has been linked in some studies to cancer.

- *Radon*—a naturally occurring radioactive gas that may be present in as many as 10% of American homes. This colorless, odorless gas is produced when uranium found in rock and soil breaks down, and it enters homes and other buildings through cracks in their foundations, walls, drains and other openings. Radon can cause serious lung damage if inhaled and is the second leading cause of lung cancer after smoking.

- *Tobacco smoke*—from cigarettes, pipes, etc. Approximately 467,000 tons of tobacco are burned indoors every year, making tobacco smoke the most common indoor pollutant. It contains more than 4,000 chemicals, including 200 known poisons and 50 cancer-causing substances. Secondhand smoke has been linked to numerous health problems, including lung cancer, nasal sinus cancer, heart disease, respiratory tract infections, asthma, ear infections and sudden infant death syndrome (SIDS).

- *Lead*—a component of paint in most houses built before 1950. However, the U.S. Department of Housing and Urban Development (HUD) suspects that 74% of all homes that were built before 1980 have some amount of lead paint on their walls. If lead dust is inhaled, it can cause significant damage to cells and tissues and lead to a host of health problems.

- *Biological pollutants*—molds, mildew, bacteria, fecal droppings from dust mites and other insects, animal dander and viruses. These can be in the air we breathe either alone or attached to particles of dust. In fact, more than 40,000 dust mites can be found in just one ounce of dust. These biological pollutants are linked to household allergies and asthma.

Indoor air pollution has been estimated to be responsible for or aggravate half of all illnesses, including:

- Respiratory infections
- Asthma
- Toxic and allergic reactions
- Mucous membrane irritation
- Nervous system effects
- Cardiovascular effects
- Reproductive effects
- Lung cancer
- Headaches
- Dry eyes
- Nasal congestion
- Nausea
- Fatigue

Breathe Easy: How to Make Your Home Safer with Cleaner Air

Once you understand the dangers associated with indoor air pollution, keeping the air in your home as pure as possible becomes a huge priority. Fortunately, significantly improving your home's air quality isn't all that difficult. The Environmental Protection Agency recommends a three-pronged approach.

Strategy 1: Source Control

Sometimes the best way to reduce or eliminate indoor air pollution is to cut it off at the source. This is a simple way to eliminate pollutants like tobacco smoke from your home. If you don't feel like you can quit smoking completely, another method of source control is to only smoke outside and to ask everyone else to do the same.

Other methods of source control include:

- Test the air in your home for radon and address any potential problems as soon as possible.
- Keep the humidity in your home as low as possible by using a dehumidifier. This will help fight mold, mildew, dust mites and other biological pollutants. If you think you already have a problem with these pests, try to eliminate them with non-chemical methods rather than harsh sprays.
- Make sure that your furnace, chimney and other heating systems are running cleanly and efficiently.
- Check the labels on all of your cleaning products. If it says not to use the product in an enclosed space—don't do it. You can also look for "natural," "green" or "organic" cleaning products at your local health food store or supermarket.
- Only buy and use furniture that is made of solid wood. Pressed wood, like particleboard and plywood, can release formaldehyde into the air for years after it is brought into your home.

Strategy 2: Improve Ventilation

Airtight, insulated living spaces are great for conserving energy (and heat) in the winter months, but they trap pollutants and allow them to accumulate. An easy way to combat this is to air out your house frequently. Open up your windows and doors the next time the weather is good to bring in fresh air and let out contaminated air. Other great ways to improve ventilation are to use fans to increase circulation and use the ventilators in your bathroom and kitchen regularly.

Simple Tips for Improving the Air Quality in Your Home

- Crack a window or a door each day to let in fresh air
- Use nontoxic household cleaning products—a gallon of water mixed with 1/4 cup of white vinegar and a teaspoon of baking soda makes a good all-purpose cleaner. You can also check at your local natural foods store or supermarket for products that are biodegradable and free of phosphates, petroleum, hydrochloric acid, sulfuric acid, benzene and chlorine
- Keep your furnace, dehumidifier, air conditioner and air ducts clean, and change all filters frequently
- Test for radon and lead
- Decorate with lots of live plants—plants absorb carbon dioxide and release oxygen. Plus, plants like the Rubber Plant, Dracaena, English Ivy, Ficus Alii, Boston Fern, Peace Lily, Corn Plant, Golden Pothos, Florist's Mum, Gerbera Daisy, Spider Plants and a number of palms have a very high rating for removing formaldehyde and neutralizing other airborne toxins

---

Strategy 3: Air Purification

No matter how hard you try, you can't eliminate all sources of pollution in your home, and ventilation can only do so much. Therefore, there will always be some level of air pollution in your home. However, there is a way to minimize the number of unhealthy particles floating around and diminish the health risks that they bring—air purification systems. Things like air filters and ionizers can handle pollution that you, by yourself, could never hope to eliminate, decreasing the concentration of indoor air pollutants by at least 80%.

Air Filters

Air filters are an effective way to remove particles like dust, pollen, some molds, animal dander, dust mites and cockroach body parts and droppings from the air. Since many of these particles are associated with asthma and allergy symptoms, air filters are often recommended for people affected by these conditions. While even the most advanced air purification systems cannot eliminate all airborne irritants, especially the ones released when a person comes in contact with things like pillows, rugs and furniture, they can help improve respiratory health.

For example, research presented in *The New England Journal of Medicine* in 2004 showed that while adding air filters to the homes of children with asthma did not completely alleviate their asthma symptoms, the purified air did help and it created an overall healthier environment. For every 2-week period during the yearlong study, the children living in homes with filters had fewer days with asthma symptoms than the group living without filters, and this trend continued during the year following the study.

Most Common Types of Air Filters for Home Use

- *High Efficiency Particle Air (HEPA) Filters*—made up of a mat of randomly arranged fibers that capture a minimum of 99.97% of airborne particles (up to 0.3 microns in diameter). They must be replaced every 6 months to a year to be effective, but will not help filter particles that have already settled onto surfaces
- *Electrostatic Filters*—use electrical charges to attract all allergens from the airstream and collect them on electrostatic plates. These plates must be cleaned frequently to remain effective. The downside of this type of filter is that they may produce small amounts of ozone, which is an irritant in its own right.
- *Hybrid Filters*—combine the particle-reducing power of HEPA filters with materials like activated carbon, which filters gasses. Together they boost the amount of pollutants removed from the air.

Air filters are not just beneficial for people with respiratory problems, though. A study published in the *American Journal of Respiratory and Critical Care Medicine* in 2008 showed that using HEPA filters for just two days could significantly improve cardiovascular health in healthy, nonsmoking elderly adults. According to the researchers, the HEPA filters removed about 60% of the ultrafine, fine and coarse particles from the air in the participants' homes and was linked to a significant improvement in the function of small blood vessels in their fingers. While this may not sound all that exciting and/or important, this improvement in microvascular function (MVF) actually indicates an overall improvement in the function of the inner lining of all small vessels. "This suggests that indoor air filtration represents a feasible means of reducing cardiovascular risk," said Dr. Steffen Loft from the Institute of Public Health in Copenhagen. I recommend IQAir Air Purifier Filters (http://www.iqair.com/).

Healing Under Pressure: The Amazing Health Benefits of Hyperbaric Oxygen Therapy

While breathing clean air has a huge impact on our health and wellbeing, pure oxygen also has its place in the treatment and prevention of a number of serious conditions and diseases.

Hyperbaric oxygen therapy involves breathing pure oxygen in a pressurized room or chamber. During hyperbaric oxygen therapy, the air pressure can be up to three times higher than normal air pressure. Under these conditions, your lungs can absorb up to three times more oxygen than they could even if your were breathing pure oxygen at normal air pressure.

Why is this extra oxygen important? Well, as you know, all of the tissues and cells in your body need oxygen to function. But when any tissue is damaged (due to a disease or injury), it needs even more oxygen in order to survive. Since hyperbaric oxygen therapy increases the amount of oxygen your blood can carry, it promotes healing and helps fight off infections.

> **Did You Know?** Celebrities like Michael Jackson and athletic superstars like Terrell Owens and Tim Tebow have used hyperbaric oxygen chambers (and even installed them in their homes) to improve their health, slow down aging and get them back in the game.

Hyperbaric oxygen therapy is a well-established and recommended treatment for a number of conditions:

- Carbon monoxide poisoning
- Serious infections
- Wounds that won't heal
- Gangrene
- Skin or bone infection that causes tissue death
- Burns
- Severe anemia
- Abscess (collection of pus) in the brain or head

Hyperbaric oxygen therapy is also used as an alternative treatment for a number of other conditions that are caused or aggravated by reduced levels of oxygen.

Autism Spectrum Disorder (ASD)

Approximately one in every 150 children in the United States have been diagnosed with Autism Spectrum Disorder (ASD), and that number is growing at an alarming rate. This has prompted a flurry of research activity into studying the cause and treatment of this epidemic disorder. In recent years, experts have discovered that hyperbaric oxygen therapy may be an effective way to improve many autism symptoms by reducing inflammation and excess swelling in the brain tissue, increasing the amount of blood flow and oxygen the brain receives, and stimulating brain function. According to these doctors, all of these effects allow the brain to do its job better, which can improve many of the classic symptoms of ASD, including repetitive and self-stimulatory behaviors, as well as difficulties with communication, sensory perception and social interaction.

A high-quality clinical study of 62 children conducted in 2009 found that those who received 40 hours of hyperbaric oxygen therapy a month were less irritable, more responsive when people spoke to them, made more eye contact and were more sociable than kids who did not receive the treatment. They were also less sensitive to experiencing a kind of sensory overload from loud sounds and background noise. However, the greatest improvements were observed in children over the age of five with milder ASD.

Holding Back the Waves of Time: Anti-Aging Benefits

Hyperbaric oxygen therapy is often used as an anti-aging treatment to help people look and feel younger. One of the most important goals of any anti-aging therapy is to restore brain function, which often diminishes with age. If you have ever forgotten where you put your keys or realized you can't remember a friend's name, you know what I mean. Oftentimes this age-related cognitive decline is linked to a lack of oxygen and blood flow to the brain. And in time, this decreased neurological function can lead to premature aging and dementia. However, a number of studies conducted over the past three decades have shown that the "premature aging wounds" linked to decreased blood flow and oxygen absorption can be repaired with hyperbaric oxygen therapy, which leads to significant improvements in neurological, cognitive, behavioral and emotional function.

Hyperbaric oxygen therapy is not just for the brain though; it works from the inside out in other ways to help you look and feel younger. For example, hyperbaric oxygen therapy has been shown to promote the growth of new blood vessels, improve collagen formation (the substance that makes your skin look firm and youthful) and increase the amount of circulating stem cells in your blood, which benefits almost every organ in your body—including your skin!

Anti-Aging Benefits of Hyperbaric Oxygen

- Youthful, radiant skin
- Increased energy and mental focus
- Boosts your immune system
- Improves your joints, heart and vision
- Reduces age-related conditions, including strokes, heart attacks, dementia and arthritis

---

Healing the Body's Electrical System: The Key to Living a Longer, Healthier, Pain-Free Life

While what you take into your body (in the form of food, water, oxygen) is vitally important for maintaining your health and preventing disease, the root of good health lies in your nervous system. Everything you do, from breathing to reading the words on this page, happens because of electrical signals running through your body. All of these signals are produced by the internal generator we each have encased in our skulls—our brains. They are then sent down through the power lines of the body—the spinal cord and nervous system. From the time you were developing in your mother's womb until the day you die, this electrical flow controls all of your body's functions and healing processes. This is literally the power supply of life.

Knowing how significant and intricate the electrical system intertwined within our body is, you can see why it is protected by a well-built, bony structure like the spine. In fact, your brain, spinal cord and nerves are the only things in the body that are protected by bone.

The spine is made up of 24 vertebrae, or spinal bones. Each of these bones is stacked one on top of the other and attached by a joint. In this way, your spine forms a hollow column that surrounds and protects your spinal nerves from three kinds of stress (physical, chemical and emotional) and allows them to connect your brain to every other organ in your body. This free flow of "power" across your nerve system is absolutely essential for health.

> **Did You Know:** The primary function of the brain is not making decisions, processing language or even storing and recalling memories. It is maintaining your health.

Think of the nerves and the spine as the power panel box in your house. When all of the switches (breakers) are on, there is light and power in every room. But if one of these switches gets flipped, the power goes off in the corresponding section of your house. The same happens in your body if one or more of your vertebra becomes misaligned due to trauma or repetitive stress to the spine. The bone pinches the nerve, effectively flipping the switch and impeding the nerve supply to one or more of your organs, short-circuiting its function. This is known as a subluxation and is an underlying cause of many of the physical and mental disorders that are so common in our modern society.

Subluxations Are an Underlying Cause of Disease

The word "subluxation" comes from the Latin words *luxare*, which means "to dislocate," and *sub*, which means "somewhat or slightly." The World Health Organization definition of the chiropractic vertebral subluxation is:

"A lesion or dysfunction in a joint or motion segment in which alignment, movement integrity and/or physiological function are altered, although contact between joint surfaces remains intact. It is essentially a functional entity, which may influence biomechanical and neural (brain, spinal cord and nerves) integrity."

These misalignments may put pressure on or irritate the nerves that branch off from the spinal cord between each of the vertebrae and interfere with the signals traveling from the brain. Because these misalignments cause a number of different physical and chemical changes in the spine and throughout the body, chiropractors often talk about "Vertebral Subluxation Complex" or "VSC" for short.

The Five Components of Vertebral Subluxation Complexes (VSCs)

1. *Bone (osseous) Component*—the changes occurring in the vertebrae. This could mean that the vertebra is out of position (misaligned), not moving correctly or undergoing physical changes like degeneration and arthritis.
2. *Nerve Component*—malfunctioning of the nerve. Research has shown that only a small amount of pressure on the nerves in the spine can have a huge impact on their function.
3. *Muscle Component*—these affect and are affected by the VSC. Since the muscles help hold the vertebrae in place, and since nerves control the muscles, muscles play an important role in any VSC.

---

4. *Soft Tissue Component*—changes in the tendons, ligaments, blood supply and other tissues. These changes can occur in the tissue surrounding the misaligned vertebrae or far from it, at the end point of the affected nerves in organs like the heart, liver or kidneys.

5. *Chemical Component*—chemical changes triggered by the rest of the other four VSC components. These chemical changes can be slight or massive depending on which parts of the body are affected.

So what can cause subluxations to develop? Many spinal displacements come from past traumas like a fall, sports injuries, car accidents and even from birthing children. However, more and more, subluxations are being caused by the cumulative stresses of everyday life. Poor posture, improper sleeping conditions or habits, sitting at a computer or in a car all day, incorrect lifting practices, obesity and a lack of rest and exercise added together over time can lead to subluxations.

No matter how they occur, subluxations have the same effect—dysfunction. Imagine that panel box again. If you interfere with the signals traveling through your nerves, parts of your body will not get the "power" they need and will not be able to function at 100%. In other words, some part of your body will not be working properly.

> "Better than 90% of the energy output of the brain is used in relating the physical body in its gravitational field. The more mechanically distorted a person is, the less energy is available for thinking, metabolism and healing."
>
> —Dr. Roger Sperry,
> 1980 Nobel Prize for brain research

Studies at the University of Colorado have shown that as small of a misalignment as a 1/2-inch hip pull can cause at least three major stress areas in the spine. Within 20 minutes of developing, these stress areas can negatively alter nerve activity by more than 60%. As a result, the organs and body parts supplied by these damaged nerves are severely affected. Also, within 2 hours, the nerves involved rupture and begin releasing a neurotoxin that ultimately causes irreversible bone degeneration at the site of pressure. As scary as this sounds, the damage done to the body only increases if the nerve is pinched more severely.

So how does this present itself in the body? Well it depends on which vertebrae and nerves are involved. Let's say you have a subluxation that is pressing on the nerve that goes to stomach. This misalignment flips the nerve's switch, disrupting communication between the brain and stomach. Consequently, when you eat a meal your stomach won't produce enough acid because it will only receive part of the brain's instructions. This means that the food you've just eaten won't be completely digested, causing it to back up in your system. The longer it sits there the more toxic it becomes. Of course, when something toxic sits in your stomach, your body's first reaction is to get rid of it. But once again, because of the miscommunication from your brain, your body only throws it up part way, causing what we called heartburn or acid reflux.

The Importance of Posture

Research indicates that poor posture can take away 14 years of your lifespan. This is because your posture has an effect on everything in your body, from breathing to hormonal production. Therefore, improving your posture can improve:

- Spinal pain
- Headaches
- Mood
- Blood pressure
- Lung capacity

A Real Life Example—Florence K.

"Many people have noticed an improvement in my posture. Before I had my treatments my posture leaned to the right and my head bent to the right. Naturally my right shoulder drooped way down. Now my shoulders are even. Also I had trouble with my right leg. Throughout the day the upper part of my right leg would burn and prickle. That is rare now thanks to Dr. Joseph and the great staff that is here."

Not a Happy Birth Day: How Birth Trauma Can Lead to Serious Infant Health Issues

Although a large percentage of people don't notice the negative effects of subluxations until well into adulthood, many times the damage is the result of usual spinal stress that occurs during or shortly after birth. For most of us, these misalignments result in take-it-for-granted problems that build up over a period of 40, 50 or 60 years; however, subluxations have been found to be a significant cause of pain, distress and even death in young infants.

In an unpublished presentation to the American Association of Pathology and Bacteriology, Dr. Abraham Towbin implicated spinal cord injury and vertebral subluxation in 88% of cases of Sudden Infant Death Syndrome (SIDS). During or shortly after birth the neck of an infant can be injured and in some cases, broken. If the neck is broken completely, the child will be "stillborn." However, if the neck is broken in a less severe way, the child can live for days or even weeks before, for no apparent reason, he or she dies. That's what has been termed SIDS.

Subluxation occurring during or after birth has also been linked to another condition of previously unknown origin—infantile colic. Infantile colic is defined as persistent, often violent, crying for no apparent reason in otherwise healthy and thriving infants. Colic usually begins between 1 and 4 weeks following birth and usually ends spontaneously around 3 to 4 months of age. In the meantime, this distressed behavior, generally believed to be a reaction to pain, causes uncontrollable crying for many hours, day and night. It is different from normal crying because the distress does not stop when the infant's needs are met. As a result, it can be destructive to both the infant and the family.

The onset of colic follows the trauma of birth and the change to a weight-bearing environment and many colicky infants have abnormalities in their cervical and thoracic spinal joint function. Therefore chiropractors have determined that infantile colic may be caused by spinal dysfunction or subluxation and many have achieved excellent results with chiropractic adjustments for many years. In a clinical study conducted in Denmark, the researchers found that chiropractic treatment provided almost instant benefits for colicky infants. The number of hours of colic was cut in half within the first day following treatment. After 2 weeks and an average number of 3 treatments, there was a success rate of 94%. Colic stopped completely in 60% of the infants and improved greatly in 34%. No adverse side effects were reported.

> "Interference to the nervous system results in permanent damage in a short period of time and therefore, chiropractic care should begin at birth on a preventative basis."
>
> —Dr. Arpad de Nagy, Rockefeller Institute

Well-Adjusted: The Proven Benefits of Chiropractic Treatment

Most of us are tied to medical ideas that are incorrect. If we are sick or in pain we go to a doctor. And what do we expect in return? That's right, a pill. And if that doesn't work, where do we turn? To surgeons who cut us up and piece us back together. But medical treatments, especially drug and surgical treatments, have relatively little to do with fundamentally fixing what is making us ill.

Even under the best of circumstances the chances of a medical doctor finding whatever is making you ill and diagnosing it correctly are about 1 in 5. This is because a medical diagnosis has traditionally focused on naming symptoms, not determining their cause. In reality, a diagnosis that does not reveal the underlying cause of a problem is only half a diagnosis!

"69% of all diagnoses done in the country are wrong."
—Dr. C. Everett Coop, Surgeon General of the United
States

The standard "problem-oriented management approach" generally results in the use of multiple drugs that fall short of treating the true cause of illness. This is because the true cause of disease can only be uncovered when you are seen as an energy being. Dr. Richard Gerber noted that certain "energy-filled patterns" within the body seem to precede the onset of illness. According to his book *Vibrational Medicine*: "We are multidimensional beings of energy and light, whose physical body is but a single component of a larger dynamic system. The ultimate approach to healing will be to remove the abnormalities at the subtle energy level which led to the manifestation of the illness in the first place." That's what chiropractic does.'

Real Life Examples

Barbara A.—"I began chiropractic because I had no energy or motivation to do any of the daily activities I once did. I am so grateful for Joseph Family Chiropractic and the Doctors here for restoring my life to the way it should be! I feel alive again!"

David D.—"I have had spinal curvature problems for many years. This is my first time trying chiropractic, and I'm finally seeing changes! There are no side effects with chiropractic, and it helps me to be more positive! I love coming here!"

The Keys to Health Lie Within Us, Not a Pill Bottle

A pharmacist in the United States fills approximately 200-300 prescriptions a day. That's because the average American is taking about 12 different drugs. But do these drugs really do anything to improve your health? To answer that question, let's use the example of high blood pressure.

In my practice, the average patient is taking three different medications to control their blood pressure. While this medication can do a good job achieving the end result, lowering blood pressure, if a patient stops taking his blood pressure medication, his blood pressure would go back up to where it 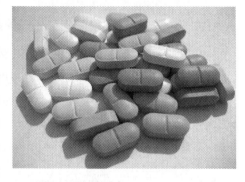 was before he started taking the medication. Does this sound like a cure to you? No. That's because the drugs are targeting the symptom—high blood pressure—rather than the underlying problem. But what is the underlying problem?

Let's suppose when this patient was 15 years old he tripped and fell, causing one of his vertebra to go out of alignment. Maybe he felt some pain, or maybe he didn't. Either way, this misaligned vertebra started pressing on the nerve that controls blood pressure (typically C1). So what will happen if the nerve supply that controls blood pressure is altered or slowed. That's right, your blood pressure goes up. So while blood pressure medicine may help for a while, a better way to truly deal with high blood pressure is to realign the spine, taking the pressure off the nerve and allowing the electric current to flow freely again. A study done at Rush University in Chicago showed that restoring correct spinal alignment (via chiropractic adjustments to the "Atlas" vertebra) reduced blood pressure to normal levels, which is the same reduction seen in patients taking two blood pressure medications.

A Real Life Example—Evelyn B.

"I have been to many doctors over the last 25 years seeking treatment for various problems after being involved in an automobile accident. After a while the doctors sent me to a psychiatrist. After two very expensive sessions I decided to go to a chiropractor. It has helped with my blood pressure, back pain, leg pain, and headaches ALL WITHOUT MEDICATION!! I have a heart condition (A FIB) and it has also helped in that area. We are continuing treatment for this condition and looking ahead to a reduction in my heart medications as well. I tell everyone I know about the benefits of chiropractic care. I even bring my great granddaughters. You cannot start too soon!"

This is the fundamental difference between the approaches taken by orthodox Western medicine and chiropractors. Orthodox medicine concentrates on treating symptoms with prescriptions, while chiropractors focus on restoring the body's ability to regulate and heal itself through a healthy, functioning nerve supply. This is why chiropractors have such success treating conditions ranging from headaches and chronic pain to fertility issues, asthma and ear infections.

A Real Life Example—Courtney W.

"I would have never thought my acne could be helped by chiropractic. Thank God I tried it because not only have I seen changes in my acne, but my allergies are better and my neck and back pain are nearly gone! You can only imagine my excitement when these changes began. I am thankful for the blessing of the Doctors at Joseph Family Chiropractic. Thank you for all you have done for my family and me!"

"Orthodox medicine tends to treat the symptom and once it has made the symptom go away, it tells the patient that his or her condition is cured or at least controlled. Actually, in most cases, the disease hasn't been treated at all. Its symptoms have been masked or obliterated, but in due time the disease may well assert itself in another direction."

—Dr. Robert C. Atkins,
Creator of the Atkins Diet

A Real Life Example—Eleanor H.

"I have had arthritis for many years but suffered with it. I took Tylenol and aspirin until I became allergic to the Tylenol. By 1997 I could not even walk and finally gave in to a wheelchair. My orthopedic surgeon diagnosed me with "bone on bone" in my knees. This started a long history of surgery stories: 2 knees, 2 hips, hysterectomy, gall bladder, and hernia. I was still in severe pain in my lower back. I was diagnosed with my sciatica being severely inflamed. I was given epidurals and when they stopped working there was talk of a neurosurgeon.

I was petrified! I prayed and prayed. A few Sundays later a friend who sat next to me in church shared her story. She had sciatica and saw Dr. Joseph. With my body still racked with pain and medications, I decided to go and meet him.

He was young, charismatic, and very informative, and I needed some relief from this pain and medication. So I agreed to his program and made a commitment to myself and him.

My healing began! X-rays and treatment. Yes! Not without pain but WITHOUT medication. I began to think clearer. After each treatment I seemed a little better.

Gradually after five weeks I AM PAIN FREE!!! Dr. Joseph says we take better care of our cars than we do our bodies. We need the maintenance too."

Low Back Pain

One of the most common complaints seen by most chiropractors, including myself, is low back pain. Low back pain affects at least 31 million Americans at any time and is one of the most common reasons for missed work. While many people turn to pain relievers and bed rest to try to treat the symptoms, chiropractic spinal adjustments are a safe and effective spine pain treatment. In fact, several extensive reviews of the available scientific research have shown that chiropractic adjustments are safer, more effective and more cost-effective than medical management of low back pain, causing the Agency for Health Care Policy and Research to recommend spinal adjustment as the only safe and effective, drugless form of initial professional treatment for acute low back problems in adults.

> **Real Life Examples**
>
> **Gloria M.**—"I have been experiencing back, leg and neck pain for 30 years. No medical doctor has been able to help me. I finally gave chiropractic a try. I have already begun to see changes! My back pain is much better! I am excited to continue and look forward to seeing more changes!"
>
> **Donna R.**—"I have suffered for several years from neck and back pain. It had escalated to a point where my extremities were being compromised. I had numbness, shooting pain and lack of motor control in both arms and legs. Since chiropractic care most of the numbness and extremity pain has subsided and I have more mobility in my neck. Conventional medicine did very little for any corrective aspects and all of the medicine made me worse in other ways. Natural chiropractic care has been the best solution for me."

Pregnancy

Chiropractic treatment is also very important for pregnant women, especially because of the risk that medications, both prescription and over-the-counter, pose to the growing fetus. There is no such thing as a safe drug, as it is pretty much impossible to find any drug that has not been linked to birth defects in laboratory animals. Even antibiotics like tetracycline, aspirin, cough syrup and cold and flu medications have been linked to fetal damage and miscarriage in humans.

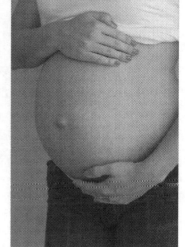

Did You Know? The total number of deaths caused by conventional medicine is an astounding 783,936 per year, making the American medical system the leading cause of death and injury in the US.

Benefits of Chiropractic Care During Pregnancy

- May help maintain pregnancy
- Controls vomiting
- Relieves back pain
- Normalizes body functions in women with conditions such as preeclampsia (high blood pressure)
- Helps control premature contractions
- Eases back labor
- Assists in delivering full-term infants, shortening labor by 50-60% and lessening the need for medication by at least 50%
- Can correct breech presentations in which the baby isn't positioned properly for birth
- Reduces the risk of developing postpartum depression

A Real Life Example—Barbara O.

"I came in because I was experiencing headaches, as well as numbness in my hands during my pregnancy. Thanks to the chiropractic adjustments given by the doctors here at Joseph Family Chiropractic, I now have less of both and I am feeling great!"

Choosing a Chiropractor

While the philosophy that chiropractic treatment is based on has never changed, some chiropractors have changed for greater social acceptance. Consequently, there are now two different types of chiropractors: musculoskeletal chiropractors who work on symptom relief and traditional wellness chiropractors who work on subluxation and structural correction.

Symptom-Relief Chiropractors

Like the typical medical doctor, this type of chiropractor primarily focuses on relieving symptoms, such as low back pain, headaches, etc. Adjustments are done to the spine to decompress the joints, free fixations and reduce pain. The length of treatment and frequency of adjustments are usually dictated by the patient's symptoms or insurance coverage. This usually equates to a shorter overall treatment time but still leaves the patient far short of correcting the actual cause of symptoms. As a result, the patient may feel better temporarily, but since the spine remains structurally misaligned, it degenerates silently over time and results in further damage and dysfunction to discs, joints and whatever part of the body the nerve supplies.

The Bottom Line: By only treating the symptoms, the cause remains uncorrected.

Traditional Wellness Chiropractors

This type of chiropractor focuses on the underlying causes of pain and other conditions—subluxation. Although a traditional wellness chiropractor also wants his or her patients to feel better quickly, his or her primary goal is to correct any nerve interference (subluxation) by realigning the spine to its most stable biomechanical position. The length of correction and frequency of adjustments is determined by the severity of the patient's subluxations and structural alignment, not their symptoms. Adjustment schedules are usually quite intense to ensure that optimal structural correction is achieved in the shortest amount of time.

> **A Real Life Example—Jane D.**
>
> "I have had poor posture, headaches and neck pain since 8th grade. All other chiropractors only offered me temporary relief, but here the Doctors have begun to correct my spine so I can finally have lasting relief! Already my headaches have greatly reduced, and I am able to be more active like I want to be!"

VACCINES

Which One of These Is Not Like the Others: Why Vaccines Do More Harm than Good

In the previous sections I have outlined the four essentials of health: food, water, oxygen and nerve supply. What you may have noticed is that some of the things that doctors and other traditional medical professionals tell you are absolutely necessary for both you and your children to be healthy are "missing." This is because many of the things traditional Western medicine counts as "essential for health" actually aren't. In fact, they may even cause and promote many of the diseases and disorders that are present in today's society at epidemic levels. The most prominent example of this is vaccines.

The debate over vaccines has been raging for hundreds of years with one side fearing the potential side effects of immunization more than

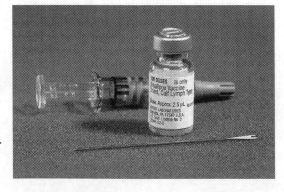

the diseases they supposedly fight, and the other side pushing for more vaccines at younger ages. With the media reporting that vaccines may or may not cause autism, autoimmune diseases and allergies while at the same time warning about viral pandemics that could kill millions without the presence of a vaccine to save us.

With such vocal opposition, deciding whether to follow the recommended immunization schedule for your children or even getting a flu shot yourself can be fraught with fear and indecision. But in my experience, I have found, like Dr. J. Anthony Morris, former Chief Vaccine Control Officer for the FDA, "There is a great deal of evidence to prove that immunization of children does more harm than good."

Most Common Reasons Parents Reject Vaccinations

- Consider vaccines dangerous and ineffective
- Prefer to promote natural rather than artificial immunity
- Already have a vaccine-injured child
- Have religious or philosophical objections to vaccination

Shots and Vaccines: Are We Playing Russian Roulette with Our Children's Health?

According to the CDC: "Children need immunizations (shots) to protect them from dangerous childhood diseases. These diseases can have serious complications and even kill children." As a result, the number of vaccinations we give our children has increased exponentially and now covers a wide-range of potentially deadly, as well as a number of non-fatal, illnesses:

- Measles
- Mumps
- Rubella
- Hepatitis A & B
- Chicken pox (*varicella zoster*)
- Polio
- Hib (*H. influenza type B*)
- Pneumococcal
- Diphtheria
- Pertussis (whooping cough)
- Tetanus
- Rotavirus
- Seasonal flu

Number of Childhood Vaccines

1950—3 vaccines (total)
2010—25 vaccines by 6 months
—36 vaccines by 18 months
—43 vaccines by 6 years
—68 vaccines by 11-12 years

But what exactly are we injecting our children with? In addition to live and killed bacteria, viruses and their toxins, children are injected with some of the most lethal poisons known to man, including:

- Formaldehyde
- Mercury
- Aluminum

- Phenol (carbolic acid)
- Borax (ant killer)
- Ethylene glycol (antifreeze)
- Dye
- Acetone (nail polish remover)
- Latex
- MSG
- Glycerol
- Polysorbate 80/20
- Sorbitol
- Monkey, cow, chick, pig, sheep and dog tissue and cells (which may be contaminated with animal viruses)
- Casein
- Human fetal cells
- Antibiotics
- Genetically modified yeast
- Animal bacterial and viral DNA (which may affect the recipient's DNA)

Some parents think that no matter what vaccines contain, guaranteeing their child's protection against contagious illnesses is worth the risk. However, despite what public health officials and doctors are constantly telling parents, vaccines don't actually do what they are advertised to do—keep children from getting sick with potentially serious diseases. Outbreaks have occurred in populations where 100% of the people have been vaccinated. In one school, 98.7% of the 137 children who contracted measles had been vaccinated!

Other studies have found that getting a pertussis (whooping cough) vaccine actually increased a child's chances of getting pertussis. In a study published in the *Journal of Infectious Diseases* in 1994, the majority of cases of whooping cough occurred in children younger than one year who had been vaccinated. Many of these children actually caught whooping cough from the vaccine! However, because of the blind faith most doctors put in these vaccinations, these children are usually diagnosed as having 'croup.'

But, unfortunately, getting whooping cough or the measles is not the worst thing that can happen as a result of vaccines. According to Dr. Robert Mendelsohn, "Immunization against relatively harmless childhood diseases may be responsible for the dramatic increase in . . . cancer, leukemia, rheumatoid arthritis, multiple sclerosis, Lou Gehrig's disease (ALS), lupus and Guillain-Barre syndrome." It is also vaccinated children that go on to develop Autism Spectrum Disorder (ASD), asthma, skin disorders, immune system disorders, neurological disorders, ADD (attention deficit disorder), ADHD (attention deficit hyperactivity disorder), other behavioral disorders, meningitis, dyslexia, hearing and vision problems, conditions that are rare in non-vaccinated children.

"Have we traded mumps and measles for cancer and leukemia?"

—Dr. Robert Mendelsohn, pediatrician and
vocal critic of the medical establishment

A Shot to the Head: Vaccines Contain Excitotoxins

If you think back to our discussion of food, you should remember the damage that excitotoxins like MSG can do to the body, especially the brain. The fact of the matter is, vaccines contain a number of even more dangerous components that promote excitotoxicity in the brain, which, when given in the current intensive schedule, can lead to serious developmental disorders like autism and even sudden infant death syndrome (SIDS).

Most of the brain is formed during the last trimester of pregnancy through the first 2 years of life. Researchers have found that much of this development is controlled by carefully timed alterations in brain glutamate levels and the activity of glutamate transporters, as well as immune system chemicals called cytokines. This 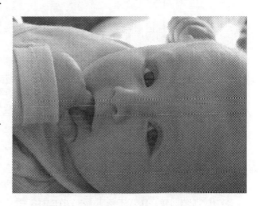 interaction between immune cytokines and glutamate helps regulate the differentiation of many types of brain cells and the development of the synaptic connections in the brain that allows information to travel from one place to another.

Because of all of the intense brain development that is taking place, the first two years of life are obviously a critical period of time for any child, and any disruptions in this process can have severe and long-term consequences. Why then do we decide to constantly stimulate the immune system with vaccines and put this entire process at risk?

Current Immunization Guidelines					
Pregnancy	*Birth*	*2 Months*	*4 Months*	*6 Months*	*1 Year*
Flu	Hep B	Hep B	DTaP	Hep B	PVC
		DTaP	PVC	DTaP	Hib
		PVC	Hib	PVC	Varicella
		Hib	Polio	Hib	Hep A
		Polio	Rabies	Polio	Flu
		Rotavirus		Rotavirus	MMR
				Flu	

When you stimulate the systemic immunity you immediately activate the brain's special immunity—within minutes. This immune system is controlled by brain cells called microglia that produce a number of different chemicals, including cytokines, chemokines, eicosanoids, proteases, complement proteins and at least two excitotoxins. While all of these chemicals can act in very positive ways in the brain under normal conditions, when they are overproduced they can be very destructive. This is what happens with childhood vaccinations.

According to Dr. Russell Blaylock, a baby's first exposure to a vaccine (usually a flu shot while he or she is still in the womb), "primes" the microglia cells. This basically sets these cells to "go" so the next time they are activated (with the Hep B vaccine at birth), they release large amounts of toxic chemicals into the brain.

Under normal circumstances, if the child had gotten sick with the flu for example, once the virus was taken care of and the child was healthy again the inflammatory responses caused by the activated microglia would go away and any of the damage caused by this reaction would be fixed. However, the closely spaced inoculation schedule doesn't allow the brain to recover before stimulating it again. To top it off, vaccines contain live viruses, contaminants and other constituents that can work their way into microglia cells and keep them constantly stimulated. This is probably one of the major underlying causes of Autism Spectrum Disorder (ASD).

Autism Spectrum Disorder (ASD)

Mercury is probably one of the best-known components of vaccines that has been linked to ASD development. While mercury is a known neurotoxin, it also increases excitotoxicity in the brain. In a series of experiments involving monkeys, researchers found that long-term exposure to very small amounts of methylmercury caused extensive microglia activation that lasted for 6 months after the last dose of mercury. They also demonstrated that the methylmercury was converted to ionic mercury (Hg^+) in the body and was distributed into the brain. This is alarming for two reasons, firstly ionic mercury is the most toxic form of mercury and most difficult to remove from the brain. Secondly, only 7% of methylmercury is converted to the ionic form in the brain while 34% of the ethylmercury found in vaccines is converted into its ionic form, making it much more dangerous.

Mercury is just one of the adjuvant metals found in vaccines that have been shown to activate microglia, even in minute quantities. Other include:

- Aluminum
- Fluoride and fluroaluminum complexes
- Cadmium

Aluminum adjuvants, such as aluminum phosphate, aluminum hydroxide and hydrated aluminum potassium sulfate, were first added to vaccines in 1926. While research has shown that this aluminum can remain at the site of injection for years, it also has been shown to accumulate in the brain. A group of Purdue University researchers lead by Richard Flarend injected rabbits with radiolabeled aluminum hydroxide and aluminum phosphate in a dose that was equivalent to what is found in vaccines (0.85mg). The aluminum was rapidly absorbed into the blood and entered into all of the major organs of the body, including the kidney, spleen, liver, heart, lymph nodes and brain. And this was from just *one vaccine*! Since aluminum is accumulative and children receive multiple vaccines, it builds up in the microglia, keeping them constantly activated.

There are a number of other non-metal vaccines components that can activate the brain's immune system and can lead to chronic microglia activation:

- Viral and bacterial contaminants (including DNA fragments)
- Live viruses (MMR as well as polio)
- Protein additives and contaminants
- Lipopolysaccharide (LPS)
- MSG

In 2001, it was shown for the first time that injecting the lipopolysaccharide (LPS) found in vaccines decreases learning in mice. While the injections did not noticeably damage the neurons, it significantly impaired both spatial and associative learning. LPS injection also elevated immune cytokine (IL-1) levels, which has been shown to alter the levels of norepinephrine and serotonin in the hippocampus. Impaired learning and elevated serotonin levels have both been described in ASD.

Sudden Infant Death Syndrome (SIDS)

Excitotoxicity and chronic brain inflammation may also explain the elusive causative link between vaccinations and sudden infant death syndrome (SIDS). In 1986, pediatric researchers studying SIDS believed babies were dying because of an inborn fault in the breathing control center in their brains. However, there is a very high concentration of microglia cells in the brain stem, which controls breathing and cardiovascular function, so chronic activation of these cells triggered by vaccines is a more likely scenario.

> "My suspicion, which is shared by others in my profession, is that the nearly 10,000 SIDS deaths that occur in the United States each year are related to one or more of the vaccines that are routinely given children. The pertussis vaccine is the most likely villain, but it could also be one or more of the others."
>
> —Dr. Robert Mendelsohn

Viera Scheibner, one of the foremost researchers of vaccine dangers and vaccine inefficacy, started her research in the mid-1980s. In one of her first experiments, a baby's breathing was monitored for more than three weeks without any issues. Then suddenly, one day after being vaccinated, the mother recorded a series of alarms warning that her child was under stress because his breathing was shallow (hypopneas) or had stopped temporarily (apneas).

A non-stop, hour-by-hour recording of the baby's breathing while he was in his crib showed increased stress patterns after he received his vaccinations. For instance, after the baby was given his third triple antigen shot (DPT—diphtheria, pertussis, tetanus) his breathing changed significantly, producing peaks in the graph indicating increased stress levels.

Scheibner later found that this wasn't an isolated case. While there were individual differences, and some children reacted more than others, the pattern of stressed breathing following vaccination was the same. The graphs showed a number of days with no stressed breathing. Then the child is vaccinated (day zero), and within one hour, the baby's stress level begins to go up and down. In all cases there was a 48-hour reaction after vaccination with a flare-up. Then the stress level went down during the next few days until there was another stress flare-up around days five to seven. The stress level again went down before another flare-up at day 16. After the stress level went down again, there was only a slight increase in the stress level towards the 24th day.

Even babies whose mothers reported no fevers or crying had slightly increased stress levels on the same critical days as those babies who had stronger reactions. According to Scheibner's reports, two out of ten randomly picked babies had to be admitted to the hospital with serious breathing problems on one of these critical days.

Forty-eight hours, five to seven days, day 16 and day 24 are not just critical days in Scheibner's experiments. In a separate study, there were 41 babies who died within 21 days of their first triple-antigen injection, and there was a clustering of these deaths along the *critical days* recorded by Scheibner. Based on this and other SIDS research, it is estimated that 95% of SIDS deaths are caused by vaccines.

Other Conditions Linked to Vaccination

Cancer	Ocular palsies
Autoimmune diseases	Deafness
Pervasive developmental disorder (PDD)	Otitis media
	Ulcerative colitis
Asperger's syndrome	Irritable bowel disease
Eczema	Crohn's disease
Meningitis	Arthritis
Encephalitis	Arthralgia (joint pain)
Guillain-Barre syndrome	Learning disorders
Convulsions and seizures	Chronic fatigue
Anaphylaxis	Diabetes
Thrombocytopenia (low platelet count)	Multiple sclerosis
Optic neuritis	Degenerative diseases of the bone and cartilage

And this list may be incomplete. According to the FDA, doctors underreport vaccination side effects and injuries by 90%. Another report revealed that only 1 in every 50 children injured by a vaccine (just 2%) is ever reported. This may be because doctors refuse to acknowledge that such reactions are inherent to vaccinations. After all, they were taught in medical school that vaccines are very safe.

"The only safe vaccine is one that is never used."
—Dr. James R. Shannon, former Director of the
National Institutes of Health

Is It Possible to Say No?

We are told our children will not be able to attend school without all of the mandatory vaccines. But this is simply **not true**! Under the Constitution, parents still have the final say as to what can be put into their children's bodies. Therefore, almost every state (except Mississippi and West Virginia) have exemptions that allow children who do not have all of their vaccinations to get into school.

These exemptions can include:

- *Medical*—Must be authorized by a doctor. If your child has asthma, diabetes, seizure disorders or any other chronic immune disease, all of the information from the pharmaceutical companies says that vaccines are contraindicated and should not be administered. However, most doctors pay this little attention and continue to vaccinate, making this exemption nearly impossible to attain.
- *Religious*—If you believe we were made perfect and vaccines tamper with that perfection. Some school or health personnel may say that religious objections only pertain to certain specified religious groups, but this is *untrue.*
- *Philosophical*—This is the easiest way to avoid vaccines, and it has been used successfully in many states. However, not many parents are aware of this.

Why Flu Shots Are More Dangerous than the Flu

Vaccines are not just a medical dilemma for children. Every year adults, especially the elderly, are urged to get a flu shot. According to the media, the medical establishment and the government we are facing a possible flu epidemic, the flu shot is safe and it saves lives. However, even in adults, the benefits of this vaccine definitely don't outweigh the risks.

First of all, flu shots, like their childhood vaccine counterparts, contain toxic ingredients like:

- *Mercury (thimerosal)*—one of the most poisonous substances known; has been linked to nerve damage, autism, dementia and other chronic conditions
- *Formaldehyde*—a known carcinogen linked to brain, colon, sinus, nasopharnyx and lymphatic cancers, as well as leukemia; a probable gastrointestinal, liver, immune system, nerve, reproductive system and respiratory poison
- *Antibiotics*—can cause mild to life-threatening allergic reactions
- *Egg proteins*—can cause serious allergic reactions in sensitive people; may also include avian contaminant viruses
- *Polysorbate 80*—known to cause cancer in animals
- *Monosodium glutamate (MSG)*—a potent neurotoxin that also has possible mutagenic and reproductive effects
- *Sodium deoxycholate*—damages DNA and promotes tumor growth and development
- *Triton X-100*—a strong detergent that kills sperm and can cause a wide range of side effects ranging from chills and confusion to lightheadedness and muscle aches
- *Beta propiolactone*—known to cause cancer; suspected as being a respiratory, gastrointestinal, liver, skin and sensory organ poison

There is actually 25 micrograms of mercury per dose in most flu shots. That is five times the maximum amount judged as safe by the CDC for a 110-pound person! And there is even more mercury if your doctor uses a multi-dose vial. While adults don't have to worry about this mercury leading to autism, it may contribute to the development of Alzheimer's. According to Dr. Hugh Fudenberg, the world's leading immunogeneticist, a person who has had five consecutive flu shots has a ten times higher risk of developing Alzheimer's disease, probably due to mercury-induced brain damage. And there could be more issues . . . we just don't know. The long-term consequences of repeated influenza vaccinations has never been tested.

Secondly, researchers report that studies "substantially overestimate the [flu] vaccine's benefit." A review of 48 reports that included more than 66,000 adults found that "vaccination of healthy adults only reduced the risk of influenza by 6% and reduced the number of missed work days by less than one (0.16) days. It did not change the number of people needing to go to the hospital or take time off work." In a review of 64 studies in 98 flu seasons, for the elderly living in nursing homes, "flu shots were non-significant for preventing the flu. For elderly living in the community, vaccines were not (significantly) effective against influenza, ILI or pneumonia."

Finally, the flu is not as deadly and widespread as its supporters would lead you to believe. Most people who suffer from fever, fatigue, cough and aching muscles during the winter months think they have the flu—they don't. Instead they have what is known as an "influenza-like illness" (ILI). ILIs are linked to many different germs like rhinoviruses, respiratory syncytial virus (RSV), adenoviruses, parainfluenza viruses, Legionella app., Chlahydia pneumoniae, Mycoplasma pneumoniae and Streptococcus pneumoniae but *not* the flu virus. In one study, the CDC found that only 13.4% of people who had flu symptoms actually had the flu. The rest had an ILI.

Also, the often-reported statistic that the flu kills 36,000 people every year is simply *not true*. Government statistics lump flu and pneumonia deaths together, but flu deaths make up only a small percentage of the total. In 2002 when flu plus pneumonia deaths were reported at over 60,000, only 753 were actually caused by the flu. In 2001 the total number of flu deaths were 267.

If flu isn't even a deadly disease why do we want to protect ourselves from it? It seems as though we have gotten to the point where we have become so afraid of "germs" and "illness" that we have lost sight of the fact that illness plays an important role in our lives and, perhaps surprisingly, our overall health.

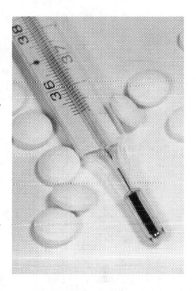

Hippocrates, the "Father of Medicine," recognized the role illness plays in the larger picture of health when he wrote: "Diseases are crises of purification, of toxin elimination. Symptoms are the natural defenses of the body. We call them diseases, but in fact they are the cure of diseases." Think about it: when we are infected with a virus like the flu we start to run a fever. Yes this causes us to feel sick and lethargic, but what is the body attempting to do? It is trying to create an environment that is much too hot for the virus to survive and reproduce. But instead of allowing our body's natural defense to do their job, what do we do? That's right, we reach for the pill bottle. But while this may make us feel better in the short term, it may actually hinder our recovery. In one study flu suffers who took aspirin or acetaminophen were sick an average of 3.5 days longer than people who did not take the drugs.

The cleansing or detoxifying aspect of illness (fever, vomiting, diarrhea, sweating) may be why getting colds, flu and infectious diseases has been linked with improved health in adulthood. Researchers have found that those who had fever-producing infectious diseases in childhood naturally lower their risk of cancer and heart disease in later life, while another study revealed that "a history of common colds or . . . influenza . . . was associated with a decreased risk of stomach, colon, rectum and ovarian cancer." Therefore, it is much better to strengthen your immune system to better fight off influenza infections than it is to attempt to prevent them with potential dangerous flu shots.

Ways to Support Your Natural Immune Function

- Get plenty of sleep
- Don't drink alcohol to excess
- Eat a diet rich in phytonutrients from a "rainbow" of vegetables
- Avoid excess sugar and processed foods
- Take a daily multi-vitamin with plenty of zinc
- Take at least 2000 IU of vitamin D3 per day—it is more important than taking vitamin C
- Your GI tract is your first line of defense against getting sick. The more good bacteria you have in your body the better equipped you are to fight off illness. Take a good probiotic with at least 50 billion colony forming units of lactobacillus and bifidobacterium species per dose
- If you start to feel sick, herbal preparations that contain Andrographis, Allicin (garlic), Elderberry and Astragalus can help if taken when symptoms begin
- If you end up on an antibiotic, take a probiotic called saccharomyces boulardii for as long as you take the antibiotic to help prevent abnormal bacteria from adhering to your intestinal wall

EPILOGUE

The Choice Is Of Course...All Yours

Dr. Deepak Chopra states, *"you acquire a new stomach lining every five days, your skin is new every five weeks, your skeleton, seemingly so solid and rigid, is entirely new every three months. You appear to be the same outwardly, yet you are like a building whose bricks are constantly being replaced by new ones. Every year, fully 98% of the total number of atoms in your body are replaced—this has been confirmed by radioisotope studies at the Oak Ridge laboratories in California."*

Since this is true, we should ask the questions; why is it that so many Americans are sick and our country ranks 37th in overall health? Why do we need so many medications (average American takes 12 per day) and surgeries?

I pray that you have found some of the answers to the above questions in this book and that they have given you some hope. The tips that I have offered provide you several ways to prevent the disastrous phenomenon of overmedication, needless surgeries, years of poor health, pain and anguish. I am positive and confident that there are many other ways, things, or products that may get you well, and I am hopeful that they will be offered to people throughout the globe in order to end their pain and suffering.

What I have presented in his book is not a quick fix, a magic pill, or even a program that is one-size-fits-all. One-size-fits-all programs are just that. They are designed for everyone without the consideration that we are all unique and our genetic makeup differs from one individual to the next. What you have read are what I call "survival basics". The four things; food, water, oxygen, and nerve supply are essentially the four things that everyone must have in order to age harmoniously and prevent disease from building in our body. Without one of these four things, we'd die very quickly. However, if we interfere with any of the four, dis-ease (lack of ease) begins to build slowly over time, which is the foundation for the diseases that we all wish to avoid like cancer, heart disease, diabetes and Alzheimer's.

Don't you want to wake up every day looking forward to the next, having vibrant energy, strong, clear memory, being pain free and not looking back at when things used to be that way? No matter where you are, there is help for you. Most people simply need a helping hand. There is absolutely no reason for anyone to be trapped by his or her health. Without the proper advice and a helping hand, the wrong lifestyles will only take away your most precious asset, which is your health. Share this book with a friend or family member or let my staff and me help you. Thousands of people like you have been helped that had conditions which many of the so-called "experts" considered impossible to relieve.

May God Bless you and your journey towards achieving optimal health!

RESOURCES

Food

Pensabene JW, Fiddler W, Gates RA, Fagan JC, Wasserman. Effect of frying and other cooking conditions on nitrosopyrrolidine formation in bacon. *J Food Sci.* 1974;39(2):314-316.

Hartman PE. Review: Putative mutagens and carcinogens in foods. I. Nitrate/nitrite ingestion and gastric cancer mortality. *Environ Mutagen.* 1983;5(1):111-121.

Eichholzer M, Gutzwiller F. Dietary nitrates, nitrites, and N-nitroso compounds and cancer risk: A review of the epidemiologic evidence. *Nutr Rev.* 1998;56(4):95-105.

Shadhu MS, White IR, McPherson K. Systematic review of the prospective cohort studies on meat consumption and colorectal cancer risk: A meta-analytical approach. *Cancer Epidemiol Biomarkers Prev.* 2001;10:439.

Center for Science in the Public Interest. *Chemical cuisine: Learn about food additives.* http://www.cspinet.org/reports/chemcuisine.htm. 2001.

Ito N, Fukushima S, Tsuda H. Carcinogenicity and modification of the carcinogenic response by bha, Bht, and other antioxidants. *Clin Rev Toxicol*. 1985;15(2):109-150.

Witschi HR, Doherty DG. Butylated hydroxyanisole and lung Tumor development in A/J Mice. *Toxicol Sci*. 1984;4(5):795-801.

Parke DV, Lewis DF. Safety aspects of food preservatives. *Food Addit Contam*. 1992;9(5):561-577.

McCann D, Barrett A, Cooper A, et al. Food additives and hyperactive behaviour in 3-year-old and 8/9-year-old children in the community: a randomised, double-blinded, placebo-controlled trial. *Lancet*. 2007;370(9598):1560-1567.

Neuman W. What's inside the bun? *NY Times*. July 1, 2011. http://www.nytimes.com/2011/07/02/business/02hotdog.html

Blaylock RL. *Excitotoxins: The taste that kills*. Santa Fe, NM: Health Press; 1997.

Frieder B, Grimm VE. Prenatal monosodium glutamate causes long-lasting cholinergic and adrenergic changes in various brain regions. *J Neurochem*. 1987;48(5):1359-1365.

Blaylock RL. *Excitotoxins (MSG, aspartame)*. http://www.youtube.com/watch?v=bEh3_JBDErw. December 14, 2010.

Soffritti M, Belpoggi F, Esposti DD, Lambertini L. Aspartame induces lymphomas and leukaemias in rats. *Eur J Oncol*. 2005;10(2).

Soffritti M, Belpoggi F, Tibaldi E, Esposti DD, Lauriola M. Lifespan exposure to low doses of aspartame beginning during prenatal life increases cancer effects in rats. *Environ Health Perspect*. 2007;115(9):1293-1297.

Hu FB, Stampfer MJ, Manson JE, et al. Dietary fat intake and the risk of coronary heart disease in women. *N Engl J Med*. 1997;337:1491-1499.

DeMaria R, Meyer LA. *Dr. Bob's Trans Fat Survival Guide: Why No-Fat, Low-Fat, Trans Fat Is Killing You.* Elyria, OH: Drugless Healthcare Solutions; 2005.

Howell WH, ed. *Howell's textbook of physiology,* 14th edition. Philadelphia, PA: W. B. Saunders Company; 1940: 777.

Vasey C. *The acid-alkaline diet for optimum health.* Rochester, VT: Healing Arts Press; 1999.

Baroody TA. *Alkalize or die: Superior health through proper alkaline-acid balance.* Waynesville, NC: Holographic Health Press; 2002.

Remer T. Influence of diet on acid-base balance. *Semin Dial.* 2000;13(4):221-226.

Sellmeyer DE, Stone KL, Sebastian A, Cummings SR. A high ratio of dietary animal to vegetable protein increases the rate of bone loss and the risk of fracture in postmenopausal women. Study of Osteoporotic Fractures Research Group. *Am J Clin Nutr.* 2001;73(1):118-122.

Biradar SS, Bahagvati ST, Shegunshi B. Probiotics and antibiotics: A brief overview. *Int J Nutr Wellness.* 2005;2(1)

Reid G, Jass J, Sebulsky MT, McCormick JK. Potential uses of probiotics in clinical practice. *Clin Microbiol Rev.* 2003;16(4):658-672.

Rachman B. Unique features and application of non-animal derived enzymes. *Clin Nutr Insights.* 1997;5(10).

Water

Batmanghelidj F. *Water for Health, for Healing, for Life: You're Not Sick, You're Thirsty.* New York, NY: Warner Books, Inc., 2003.

Mayo Clinic. Dehydration. http://www.mayoclinic.com/health/dehydration/DS00561. January 7, 2011.

Batmanghelidj F. Neurotransmitter histamine: An alternative point of view. *Sci Med Simplified.* 1990;1:8-39.

Batmanghelidj F. Is cell membrane receptor protein down-regulation also a hydrodynamic phenomenon? *Sci Med Simplified.* 1991;2:32-46.

Batmanghelidj F. For the record. *Sci Med Simplified.* 1990;1:1-7.

Chan J, Knutsen SF, Blix GG, Lee JW, Fraser GE. Water, other fluids, and fatal coronary heart disease: The Adventist Health Study. *Am J Epidemiol.* 2002;155:827-833.

Michaud DS, Spiegelman D, Clinton SK, et al. Fluid intake and the risk of bladder cancer in men. *N Engl J Med.* 1999;340:1390-1397.

Natural Resources Defense Council. Bottled water: Pure drink or pure hype? http://www.nrdc.org/water/drinking/bw/bwinx.asp. March 1999.

Centers for Disease Control. National report on humane to environmental chemicals (Fourth Report).

http://www.cdc.gov/exposurereport/executive_summary.html. February 28, 2011.

Murray TJ, Maffini MV, Ucci AA, Sonnenschein C, Soto AM. Induction of mammary gland ductal hyperplasias and carcinoma in situ following fetal bisphenol A exposure. *Reproduct Toxicol.* 2006;23:383-390.

Durando M, Kass L, Piva J, et al. Prenatal bisphenol A exposure induces preneoplastic lesions in the mammary gland in wistar rats. *Environ Health Perspect.* 2007;115(1):80-86.

Wetherill YB, Petre CE, Monk KR, Puga A, Knudsen KE. The xenoestrogen bisphenol A induces inappropriate androgen receptor activation and mitogenesis in prostatic adenocarcinoma cells. *Molec Cancer Therap.* 2002;1:515-524.

Alonso-Magdalena P, Morimoto S, Ripoll C, Fuentes E, Nadal A. The estrogenic effect of bisphenol-A disrupts the pancreatic ß-cell function in vivo and induces insulin resistance. *Environ Health Perspect.* 2006;114:106-112.

Sugiura-Ogasawara M, Ozaki Y, Sonta S, Makino T, Suzumori K. Exposure to bisphenol A is associated with recurrent miscarriage. *Human Reprod.* 2005;20:2325-2329.

Takahashi O, Oishi S. Disposition of orally administered 2,2-bis(4-hydroxyphenyl) propane (bisphenol A) in pregnant rats and the placental transfer to fetuses. *Environ Health Perspect.* 2000;108:931-935.

Kubo K, Arai O, Omura M, Wantanabe R, Ogata R, Aou S. Low dose effects of bisphenol A on sexual differentiation of the brain and behavior in rats. *Neurosci Res.* 2003;45:345-356.

Masuno H, Kidani T, Sekiya K, et al. Bisphenol A in combination with insulin can accelerate the conversion of 3T3-L1 fibroblasts to adipocytes. *J Lipid Res.* 2002;3:676-684.

von Saal F, Hughes C. An extensive new literature concerning low-dose effects of bisphenol A shows the need for a new risk assessment. *Environ Health Perspect.* 2005;113(8):926-933.

Natural Resources Defense Council. Arsenic and old laws: A scientific and public health analysis of arsenic occurrence in drinking water, its health effects, and EPA's outdated arsenic tap water standard.

http://www.nrdc.org/water/drinking/arsenic/aolinx.asp. February 2000.

Commission on Life Sciences. Arsenic in drinking water. Washington, DC: National Academy Press, 1999.

Scientific American. Tapped out?: Are chlorine's beneficial effects in drinking water offset by its links to cancer?

http://www.scientificamerican.com/article.cfm?id=earth-talks-tapped-out. January 25, 2010.

President's Cancer Panel. Reducing environmental cancer risks: what we can do now.

http://deainfo.nci.nih.gov/advisory/pcp/annualReports/pcp08-09rpt/PCP_Report_08-09_508.pdf. 2009.

Tyent USA. Water for Wellness. www.tuentusa.com.

Heil DP. Acid-base balance and hydration status following consumption of mineral-based alkaline bottled water. *J Int Soc Sports Nutr.* 2010;7(1):29.

Young RO. The pH miracle for weight loss. New York, NY: Time Warner Book Group, 2005.

Tsai CF, Hsu YW, Chen WK, et al. Hepatoprotective effect of electrolyzed reduced water against carbon tetrachloride-induced liver damage in mice. *Food Chem Toxicol.* 2009;47(8):2031-2036.

Shirahata S, Kabayama S, Nakano M, et al. Electrolyzed-reduced water scavenges active oxygen species and protects DNA from oxidative damage. *Biochem Biophys Res Commun.* 1997;234(1):269-274.

Ye J, Li Y, Hamasaki T, et al. Inhibitory effect of electrolyzed reduced water on tumor angiogenesis. *Biol Pharm Bull.* 2008;31(1):19-26.

Itokawa Y. Functional water and health: Considerations regarding alkaline ionized water research results. *Japan Oral Functional Water Academics Society Journal.* 2000:22-23.

Takahashi R, Hua ZZ, Itokawa Y. Influences of alkaline ionized water on formation and maintenance of bone structure. *6th Functional Water Symposium.* 1999: 8-9.

Takahashi R, Hua ZZ, Itokawa Y. Effects of alkaline ionized water on bone formation and maintenance. *7th Functional Water Symposium.* 2000: 80-82.

Hua ZZ, Kimura M, Itokawa Y. Influence of alkaline ionized water on rat bone volume. *Functional Water Symposium.* 1995:10-11.

Wynn E, Krieg MA, Lanham-New SA, Burckhardt P. Postgraduate Symposium: Positive influence of nutritional alkalinity on bone health. *Proc Nutr Soc.* 2010;69(1):166-173.

Hayakawa T, Shimakura T, Mikasa S, Tsuge H. Physiological effects of alkaline ionized water: Influences on intestinal fermentation products and blood components *8th Functional Water Symposium.* 2001: 32-33.

Nishina M, Tominaga N, Matsushita K, De WX, Suzuki M, Suzuki M. Effects of drinking alkaline ionized water on skin structure water in the growth process of mice. *Functional Water Research.* 2002;1(1):32.

Kim MJ, Kim HK. Anti-diabetic effects of electrolyzed reduced water in streptozotocin-induced and genetic diabetic mice. *Life Sci.* 2006;79(24):2288-2292.

Li Y, Nishimura T, Teruya K, et al. Protective mechanism of reduced water against alloxan-induced pancreatic beta-cell damage: Scavenging effect against reactive oxygen species. *Cytotechnology.* 2002;40(1-3):139-149.

Kim MJ, Jung KH, Uhm YK, Leem KH, Kim HK. Preservative effect of electrolyzed reduced water on pancreatic beta-cell mass in diabetic db/db mice. *Bio Pharma Bull.* 2007;30(2):234-236.

Pittler MH, Karagülle MZ, Karagülle M, Ernst E. Spa therapy and balneotherapy for treating low back pain: meta-analysis of randomized trials. *Rheumatology.* 2006;45(7):880-884.

Guillemin F, Constant F, Collin JF, Boulange M. Short and long-term effect of spa therapy in chronic low back pain. *Rheumatology.* 1994;33(2):148-151.

Arthritis Foundation. Water exercise. http://www.arthritis.org/water-exercise.php. 2011.

Geytenbeek J. Evidence for effective hydrotherapy. *Physiotherapy.* 2002;88(9):514-529.

Hall J, Skevington S, Maddison PJ, Chapman K. A randomized and controlled trial of hydrotherapy in rheumatoid arthritis. *Arthritis Rheumatol.* 1996;9(3):206-215.

McVeigh JG, McGaughey H, Hall M, Kane P. The effectiveness of hydrotherapy in the management of fibromyalgia syndrome: a systematic review. *Rheumatol Int.* 2008;29(2):119-130.

Evcik D, Kızılay B, Gökçen E. The effects of balneotherapy on fibromyalgia patients. *Rheumatol Int.* 2002;22(2):56-59.

Buskila D, Abu-Shakra M, Neumann L, et al. Balneotherapy for fibromyalgia at the Dead Sea. *Rheumatol Int.* 2001;20(3):105-108.

Hooper PL. Hot-tub therapy for type 2 diabetes mellitus. *N Engl J Med.* 1999;341:924-925.

Matz H, Orion E, Wolf R. Balneotherapy in dermatology. *Dermatol Ther.* 2003;16(2):132-140.

Ford ES. Serum magnesium and ischaemic heart disease: findings from a national sample of US adults. *Int J Epidemiol.* 1999;28:645-651.

Peikert A, Wilimzig C, Köhne-Volland R. Prophylaxis of migraine with oral magnesium: results from a prospective, multi-center, placebo-controlled and double-blind randomized study. *Cephalalgia.* 1996;16:257-263.

Castelli S, Meossi C, Domenici R, Fontana F, Stefani G. Magnesium in the prophylaxis of primary headache and other periodic disorders in children. *Pediatr Med Chir.* 1993;15(5):481-488.

Clauw DJ, Ward K, Wilson B, Katz P, Rajan SS. Magnesium deficiency in the eosinophilia-myalgia syndrome. Report of clinical and biochemical improvement with repletion. *Arthritis Rheum.* 1994;37(9):1331-1334.

Vormann J, Worlitschek M, Goedecke T, Silver B. Supplementation with alkaline minerals reduces symptoms in patients with chronic low back pain. *J Trace Elem Med Biol.* 2001;15(2-3):179-183.

Hornyak M, Voderholzer U, Hohagen F, Berger M, Riemann D. Magnesium therapy for periodic leg movements-related insomnia and restless legs syndrome: an open pilot study. *Sleep.* 1998;21(5): 501-505.

Cohen JS. High-dose oral magnesium treatment of chronic, intractable erythromelalgia. *Ann Pharmacother.* 2002;36(2):255-260.

Oxygen

Diamond H, Diamond M. *Living Health.* New York, NY: Warner Books, 1987.

Shaw J. Clean air, longer life. *Harvard Magazine.* May-June 2009.

Pope CA 3rd, Ezzati M, Dockery DW. Fine-particulate air pollution and life expectancy in the United States. *N Engl J Med.* 2009;360:376-386

Kleiman MT. The effects of air pollution on children. http://www.aqmd.gov/forstudents/health_effects_on_children.html. Fall 2000.

Polosa R, Salvi S, Di Maria GU. Allergic susceptibility associated with diesel exhaust particle exposure: clear as mud. *Arch Environ Health.* 2002,57(3).188-193.

Nicolai T. Environmental air pollution and lung disease in children. *Monaldi Arch Chest Dis.* 1999;54(6):475-478.

Pope CA 3rd, Burnett RT, Thun MT, et al. Lung cancer, cardiopulmonary mortality, and long-term exposure to fine particulate air pollution *J Am Med Assoc.* 2002;287:1132-1141.

Jerrett M, Burnett RT, Ma R, et al. Spatial analysis of air pollution and mortality in Los Angeles. *Epidemiology.* 2005;16(6):727-736.

World Health Organization. Air quality and health. Fact sheet 313. http://www.who.int/mediacentre/factsheets/fs313/en/index.html. September 2011.

Bennett WD. Zeman KL. Deposition of fine particles in children spontaneously breathing at rest. *Inhalation Toxicol.* 1998;10:831-842.

Brauer M, Hoek G, Van Vliet P, et al. Air pollution from traffic and the development of respiratory infections and asthmatic and allergic symptoms in children. *Am J Respir Crit Care Med.* 2002;166(8):1092-1098.

Breecher MM, Linde S. Healthy homes in a toxic world. New York, NY: John Wiley and Sons, 1992.

Levenstein MK. Everyday cancer risks and how to avoid them. Garden City Park, NY: Avery Publishing Group, 1992.

American Lung Association. Poor indoor air quality poses health risk. *Breathe Easy Magazine.* Spring/Summer 2002.

Mosley RB, Greenwell DJ, Sparks LE, et al. Penetration of ambient fine particles into the indoor environment. *Aerosol Sci Technol.* 2001;34(1):127-136.

U.S. Department of Health and Human Services. The health consequences of involuntary exposure to tobacco smoke: A report of the Surgeon General. Atlanta, GA: U.S. Department of Health and Human Services, Centers for Disease Control and Prevention, Coordinating Center for Health Promotion, National Center for Chronic Disease Prevention and Health Promotion, Office on Smoking and Health. 2006.

National Institute of Environmental Health Sciences. Asthma and its environmental triggers, scientists take a practical new look at a familiar illness. Fact Sheet #9. July 1997.

Environmental Protection Agency. Residential air cleaners (Second Edition): A summary of available information.

http://www.epa.gov/iaq/pubs/residair.html. 2008.

Custovic A, Simpson A, Pahdi H, Green RM, Chapman MD, Woodcock A. Distribution, aerodynamic characteristics, and removal of the major cat allergen found in British homes. *Thorax*. 1998;53:33-38.

Morgan WJ, Crain EF, Gruchalla RS, et al. Results of a home-based environmental intervention among urban children with asthma. *N Engl J Med*. 2004;351:1068-1080.

Brauner EV, Forchhammer L, Moller P, et al. Indoor particles affect vascular function in the aged. An air filtration-based intervention study. *Am J Respir Crit Care Med*. 2008; 177:419-425.

Allen RW, Carlsten C, Karlen B, et al. An air filter intervention study of endothelial function among healthy adults in a woodsmoke-impacted community. *Am J Respir Crit Care Med*. 2011;183(9):1222-1230.

Sulman FG. The effect of air ionization, electric fields, atmospherics and other electric phenomena on man and animal. Thomas, IL. 1980.

Grinshpun SA, Adhikari A, Lee BU, et al. Indoor air pollution control through ionization. In: *Air pollution: Modeling, monitoring and management of air pollution* (Ed: C.A. Brebbia). Southampton, U.K.: WIT Press, 2004.

Lee BU, Yermakov M, Grinshpun SA. Unipolar ion emission enhances respiratory protection against fine and ultrafine particles. *Aerosol Sci*. 2004;35:1359-1368.

Lee BU, Yermakov MY, Grinshpun SA. Removal of fine and ultrafine particles from indoor air environments by the unipolar emission of ions. *Atmospher Environ*. 2004;38:4815-4823.

Mann D. Negative ions create positive vibes. http://www.webmd.com/balance/features/negative-ions-create-positive-vibes. May 6, 2002.

Terman M, Terman JS. Treatment of Seasonal Affective Disorder with a high output negative ionizer. *J Alt Complement Med*. 1995;1(1):87-92.

Reilly T, Stevenson IC. An investigation of the effects of negative air ions on responses to submaximal exercise at different times of day. *J Hum Ergol*. 1993;22(1):1-9.

Livanova LM, Levshina IP, Nozdracheva LV, Elbakidze MG, Airapetiants MG. The protective action of negative air ions in acute stress in rats with different typological behavioral characteristics. *Zh Vyssh Nerv Deiat Im I P Pavlova*. 1998;48(3):554-557.

U.S. Environmental Protection Agency. Ozone generators that are sold as air Cleaners. http://www.epa.gov/iaq/pubs/ozonegen.html. September 30, 2010.

American Thoracic Society. Oxygen therapy. http://patients.thoracic.org/information-series/en/resources/oxygen-therapy.pdf.

National Heart Lung and Blood Institute. What Is oxygen therapy? http://www.nhlbi.nih.gov/health/health-topics/topics/oxt/. January 1, 2010.

Harch PG, McCullough V. The oxygen revolution: Hyperbaric oxygen therapy: The groundbreaking new treatment for stroke, Alzheimer's, Parkinson's, arthritis, autism, learning disabilities and more. Hobart, NY: Hatherleigh Press, 2010.

Brubakk A, Neuman T. Bennett and Elliott's physiology and medicine of diving. 5th ed. Great Britain: Elsevier Science Limited, 2003.

Thom SR, Taber RL, Mendiguren II, et al. Delayed neuropsychologic sequelae after carbon monoxide poisoning: prevention by treatment with hyperbaric oxygen. *Ann Emerg Med*. 1995;25(4):474-480.

Weaver LK, Hopkins RO, Chan KJ, et al. Hyperbaric oxygen for acute carbon monoxide poisoning. *N Engl J Med*. 2002;347(14):1057-1067.

Scheinkestel CD, Bailey M, Myles PS, et al. Hyperbaric or normobaric oxygen for acute carbon monoxide poisoning: a randomised controlled clinical trial. *Med J Aust*. 1999;170(5):203-210.

Ducassé JL, Celsis P, Marc-Vergnes JP. Non-comatose patients with acute carbon monoxide poisoning: hyperbaric or normobaric oxygenation? *Undersea Hyperb Med*. 1995;22(1):9-15.

Mader JT, Brown GL, Guckian JC, et al. A mechanism for the amelioration by hyperbaric oxygen of experimental staphylococcal osteomyelitis in rabbits. *J Infect Dis*. 1980;142(6):915-922.

Park MK, Myers RA, Marzella L. Oxygen tensions and infections: modulation of microbial growth, activity of antimicrobial agents, and immunologic responses. *Clin Infect Dis*. 1992;14(3):720-740.

Mandell GL. Bactericidal activity of aerobic and anaerobic polymorphonuclear neutrophils. *Infect Immunol*. 1974;9(2):337-341.

Faglia E, Favales F, Aldeghi A, et al. Adjunctive systemic hyperbaric oxygen therapy in treatment of severe prevalently ischemic diabetic foot ulcer. A randomized study. *Diabetes Care*. 1996;19(12):1338-1343.

Doctor N, Pandya S, Supe A. Hyperbaric oxygen therapy in diabetic foot. *J Postgrad Med*. 1992;38(3):112-114.

Abidia A, Laden G, Kuhan G, et al. The role of hyperbaric oxygen therapy in ischaemic diabetic lower extremity ulcers: a double-blind randomised-controlled trial. *Eur J Vasc Endovasc Surg*. 2003;25(6):513-518.

Kalani M, Jorneskog G, Naderi N, et al. Hyperbaric oxygen (HBO) therapy in treatment of diabetic foot ulcers. Long-term follow-up. *J Diabetes Complications*. 2002;16(2):153-158.

Rogatsky GG, Shifrin EG, Mayevsky A. Optimal dosing as a necessary condition for the efficacy of hyperbaric oxygen therapy in acute ischemic stroke: a critical review. *Neurol Res.* 2003;25(1):95-98.

McNamara D. Hyperbaric oxygen therapy helps children who have chronic brain injury. *Family Practice News.* 2006;36(19):49.

Federation for Multiple Sclerosis Therapy Centers. Long term hyperbaric oxygenation (HBO) retards progression in Multiple Sclerosis patients. 2004.

Rossingnol DA, Rossignol LW. Hyperbaric oxygen therapy may improve symptoms in autistic children. *Med Hypoth.* 2006;67(2):216-228.

Rossignol DA, Rossignol LW, Smith S, et al. Hyperbaric treatment for children with autism: a multicenter, randomized, double-blind, controlled trial. *BMC Pediatr.* 2009;9:21.

Neubauer RA, Yutsis PI. New Frontiers: Anti-Aging Properties of Hyperbaric Oxygen Therapy. *Townsend Lettr Doc Pat.* 1999;192:68-69.

Thom SR, Bhopale VM, Velazquez OC, Goldstein LJ, Thom LH, Buerk DG. Stem cell mobilization by hyperbaric oxygen. *Am J Physiol Heart Circ Physiol.* 2006;290:H1378-H1386.

Nerve Supply

Becker RO, Selden G. *The Body Electric: Electromagnetism and the Foundation of Life.* New York, NY: William Morrow and Co., 1985.

Kado DM, Huang M-H, Karlamangla AS, Barrett-Connor E, Greendale GA. Hyperkyphotic posture predicts mortality in older community-dwelling men and women: A prospective study. *J Am Geriatr Soc.* 2004;52(10):1662-1667.

Lennon J, Shealy N, Cady RK. Posture and respiratory modulation of autonomic function pain and health. *AJPM*. 1994;4(1):36-39.

Illingworth RS. Infantile colic revisited. *Arch Dis Child*. 1985;60:981-985.

Gutmann G. Blocked altantal nerve syndrome in babies and infants. *Manuelle Medicia*.1987;25:5-10.

Lewit K. *Manipulative Therapy in Rehabilitation of the Locomotor System*. London, UK: Butterworth and Co. 1985:336-340.

Nilsson N. Infantile colic and chiropractic. *Eur J Chiropr*. 1985;33:624-665.

Chapman-Smith D. Infantile colic—a new study from Denmark. *Chiropr Report*. 1989;4(1):101-104.

Leach RA. *Somatoantonomic Reflux Hypothesis in The Chiropractictic Theories: A Synopsis of Scientific Research*, 2nd ed. Baltimore, MD: Williams & Wilkins; 1986.

Kunert W. Functional disorders of internal organs due to vertebral lesions. *CIBA Symposium*. 1965;13(3):85-96.

Korr IM. *The Neurobiologic Mechanisms in Manipulative Therapy*. New York, NY: Plenum Press; 1977.

Saunders BS. Research completeness and reliability of diagnosis in therapeutic practice. *J Health Hum Behav*. 1964;5:84-94.

Gerber R. *Vibrational Medicine: The #1 Handbook of Subtle-Energy Therapies*, 3rd ed. Rochester, VT: Bear & Co.; 2001.

Atkins RC. *Dr. Atkins' Health Revolution: How Complementary Medicine Can Extend Your Life*. Boston, MA: Houghton Mifflin Co.; 1989.

Bakris G, Dickholtz M Sr, Meyer PM, Kravitz G, Avery E, Miller M, Brown J, Woodfield C, Bell B. Atlas vertebra realignment and achievement of arterial pressure goal in hypertensive patients: a pilot study. *J Hum Hypertens*. 2007 May;21(5):347-52.

Jensen M, Brant-Zawadzki M, Obuchowski N, et al. Magnetic resonance imaging of the lumbar spine in people without back pain. *N Engl J Med.* 1994;331:69-116.

Manga P, Angus D, Papadopoulos C, Swan W. A study to examine the effectiveness and cost-effectiveness of chiropractic management of low-back pain. 1993. http://www.silcom.com/~dwsmith/manga.html

Stano M. A comparison of health care costs for chiropractic and medical patients. *J Manipul Physiol Therap.* 1993;16(5):89-97.

Bigos S, Bowyer O, Braen G, et al. Acute low back problems in adults. Clinical Practice Guideline No.14. AHCPR Publication No. 95-0642. Rockville, MD: Agency for Health Care Policy and Research, Public Health Service, U.S. Department of Health and Human Services, December, 1994.

Beeson PB, McDermott E, eds. *Cecil-Loeb Textbook of Medicine,* 13th ed. Philadelphia, PA: W.B. Saunders Co.; 1971:16.

UNMC study links use of nonprescription cough medicine to miscarriages, birth defects. *Pediatric Res.* 1998:1-7.

Stein K. The value of chiropractic care in cases of pregnancy. *ACA J Chiropr.* 1964:19.

Lisi AJ. Chiropractic spinal manipulation for low back pain of pregnancy: a retrospective case series. *J Midwifery Women's Health.* 2006;51:e7-10.

Brynhildsen J, hansson A, Persson A. Hammar M. Follow-up of patients with low back pain during pregnancy. *Obstetr Gynecol.* 1998;91(2):182-186.

Reynolds JP. What is the role of osteopathic manipulative therapy in obstetric care? *JAOA.* 1974:74.

Phillips C. An effective drug-free approach to premature contractions. *Int Rev Chiropr.* 1998;54(5):76-81.

Phillips C. Back labor: a possible solution for a painful situation. *ICA Rev.* 1997.

Thomas JC. The Webster Technique in a 28-year-old woman with breech presentation & subluxation. *JVSR.* 2008:1-3.

Guthrie RA, Martin RH. Effect of pressure applied to the upper thoracic (placebo) versus lumbar areas (osteopathic manipulative treatment) for inhibition of lumbar myalgia during labor. *JAOA.* 1982;82(4):247-251.

Vaccines

Centers for Disease Control and Prevention. 10 things you need to know about immunizations.
http://www.cdc.gov/vaccines/vac-gen/10-shouldknow.htm. July 6, 2010.

Centers for Disease Control and Prevention. Morbidity and mortality weekly report (MMWR). 12/29/89/38(S-9):1-18.

Davis RM, Whitman ED, Orenstein WA. A persistent outbreak of measles despite appropriate prevention and control measures. *Am J Epidemiol.* 1987;126(3):438-449.

de Melker HE, Schellekens JFP, Neppelenbroek SE, et al. Reemergence of pertussis in the highly vaccinated population of The Netherlands: observations on surveillance data. *Emerg Infect Dis.* 2000;6(4):348-357.

Mendelsohn R. *How to Raise a Healthy Child . . . In Spite of your Doctor.* Chicago, IL: Contemporary Books. 1984.

McKeever TM, Lewis SA, Smith C. Vaccination and allergic disease: A birth cohort study. *Am J Public Health.* 2004; 94(6):985-989.

Yoneyama H, Suzuki M, Fujii K, Odajima Y. The effect of DPT and BCG vaccinations on atopic disorders. *Arerugi.* 2000;49(7):585-592.

Blaylock RL. Chronic microglia activation and excitotoxicity secondary to excessive immune stimulation: Possible factors in Gulf War Syndrome and autism. *J Am Phys Surg.* 2004;9(2):46-51.

Blaylock RL. A possible central mechanism in autism spectrum disorders, part 1. *Alt Therap Health Med.* 2008;14(6):46-53.

Blaylock RL. A possible central mechanism in autism spectrum disorders, part 2: Immunoexcitotoxicity. *Alt Therap Health Med.* 2009;15(1):60-67.

Charleston JS, Body RL, Bolender RP, Mottet NK, Vahter ME, Burbacher TM. Changes in the number of astrocytes and microglia in the thalamus of the monkey Macaca fascicularis following long-term subclinical methylmercury exposure. *Neurotoxicology.* 1996;17(1):127-138.

Charleston JS, Bolender RP, Mottet NK, Body RL, Vahter ME, Burbacher TM. Increases in the number of reactive glia in the visual cortex of Macaca fascicularis following subclinical long-term methylmercury exposure. *Toxicol Appl Pharmacol.* 1994;129(2):196-106.

Flarend RE, Hem SL, White JL, et al. In vivo absorption of aluminium-containing vaccine adjuvants using 26Al. *Vaccine.* 1997;15(12-13):1314-1318.

Arai K, Matsuki N, Ikegaya Y, Nishiyama N. Deterioration of spatial learning performances in lipopolysaccharide-treated mice. *Jpn J Pharmacol.* 2001;87:95-201.

Broderick PA. Interleukin-1-alpha alters hippocampal serotonin and norepinephrine release during open-field behavior in Sprague-Dawley animals: differences from the Fawn-Hooded animal model of depression. *Prog Neuropsychopharmacol Biol Psychiatry.* 2002;26:1355-1372.

Warren RP Singh VK. Elevated serotonin levels in autism: association with the major histocompatibility complex. *Neuropsychobiology.* 1996;34:72-75.

Scheibner V. Vaccinations: Part 1—medical research on SIDS and epidemics. *Consumer Health.* 1999;22(4).

Scheibner V. *Vaccination: 100 Years of Orthodox Research Shows that Vaccines Represent a Medical Assault on the Immune System.* UK: Minerva Books. 1993.

Renne T. Measles virus infection without rash leads to disease in adult life. *Lancet.* 1985;1(8419):1-5.

Kessler D. Introducing MEDWatch. A new approach to reporting medication and device adverse effects and product problems. *J Am Med Assoc.* 1993;269(21):2765-2768.

Froeschle J. Adverse events associated with childhood vaccines, evidence hearing on causality: Washington DC. Institute of Medicine presentations. 1992;328: Appendix B.

Vaccine Information Coalition. Educate before you vaccinate. http://www.vacinfo.org/.

Fudengerg H. National Vaccine Information Center, First International Conference on Vaccination. September 1997. Arlington, VA.

Kochanek KD, Smith BL. Deaths: Preliminary data for 2002. *Natl Vital Stats Reports.* 2004;52(13).

Jefferson T, Di Pietrantonj C, Rivetti A, Bawazeer GA, Al-Ansary LA, Ferroni E. Vaccines for preventing influenza in healthy adults. *Cochrane Database Systemic Rev.* 2010 Jul 7;(7):CD001269.

Jefferson T, Di Pietrantonj C, Al-Ansary LA, Ferroni E, Thorning S, Thomas RE. Vaccines for preventing influenza in the elderly. *Cochrane Database Systemic Rev.* 2010 Feb 17;(2):CD004876.

Centers for Disease Control and Prevention. Morbidity and mortality weekly report (MMWR). 2001;50(44):984-986.

Centers for Disease Control and Prevention. Weekly report: Influenza summary update. Week ending May 19, 2007 (Week 20). http://www.cdc.gov/flu/weekly/weeklyarchives2006-2007/weekly20.htm

Simonsen L, Reichert TA, Viboud C, Blackwelder WC, Taylor RJ, Miller MA. Impact of influenza vaccination on seasonal mortality in the US elderly population. *Arch Int Med.* 2005;165:265-272.

Arias E, Smith BL. Deaths: Preliminary data for 2001. *Natl Vital Stats Reports.* 2003;51(5).

Plaisance KI, Kunaravalli S, Wasserman SS, et al. Effect of antipyretic therapy on the duration of illness in experimental influenza A, Shigella sonnei and Rickettsia rickettsii infections. *Pharmacotherapy.* 2000;20(12):1417-1422.

Albonico HU, Braker HU, Husler J. Febrile infectious childhood diseases in the history of cancer patients and matched controls. *Med Hypoth.* 1998;51(4):315-320.

Abel U, Becker N, Angerer R, et al. Common infections in the history of cancer patients and controls. *J Cancer Res Clin Oncol.* 1991;117(4):339-344.